THE LITTLE BOOK *of* Surgical Cartoons

Evgeniy E. Perelygin

Edited by Moshe Schein

i

tfm Publishing Limited, Castle Hill Barns, Harley, Shrewsbury, SY5 6LX, UK
Tel: +44 (0)1952 510061; Fax: +44 (0)1952 510192
E-mail: info@tfmpublishing.com; Web site: www.tfmpublishing.com

Editing, design & typesetting: Nikki Bramhill BSc Hons Dip Law
First edition: © 2016
Paperback   ISBN: 978-1-910079-34-8
E-book editions: 2016
ePub   ISBN: 978-1-910079-35-5
Mobi   ISBN: 978-1-910079-36-2
Web pdf   ISBN: 978-1-910079-37-9

Printed by Cambrian Printers, Llanbadarn Road, Aberystwyth, Ceredigion, SY23 3TN
Tel: +44 (0)1970 627111; Web site: www.cambrian-printers.co.uk

Contents

Preface

Most people have found the precise nature and mechanism of humor to be elusive and difficult to define precisely. Some suggest that it is the sudden revelation of the unexpected, or an exaggeration of the commonplace; others claim that it is a sense of the ridiculous in everyday events. Surgical humor is certainly all of these, but with some of its own particular characteristics.

Surgical humor is characteristically robust. It is not for prudes or the faint-hearted. In this it may have much in common with the humor of others with challenging pursuits like soldiers or airline pilots. The surgeon will emerge from the operating room, pull off their gown and gloves, and make a joke that is hilarious to his team, but which might shock a lay person. Most surgical humor is in-house. Frequently it is close to the bone, if not frankly coarse, such is the nature of the beast.

The cartoons in this book are essentially visual burlesque. The artist is Evgeniy Perelygin, a Russian surgeon, who works at the Perm Clinical Center of the Federal Medical-Biological Agency. Many say jokes have national characteristics: German jokes are no laughing matter and many Russian jokes are perennially perineal. However, the themes of the cartoons here were conceived by the Editor to satisfy international surgical taste.

In each of the following cartoons lurks the kernel of a basic surgical truth. This truth has been blown up, distorted, and exaggerated, but remains at the heart of the picture. Each picture has a legend describing the situation. This is followed by an aphorism, quote, or comment. The Editor, Moshe Schein, is a surgeon and author of many publications, some of which have contributed cartoons and comments to this book (see overleaf).

This book is essentially for surgical eyes. For those surgical eyes (forgive me), the cartoons are all cutting edge, and will have the reader in stitches.

David M. Dent

ChM FRCS (Eng) FCS(SA) FRCP&S (Glas. Hon)

Emeritus Professor of Surgery

University of Cape Town

South Africa

- *Aphorisms & Quotations for the Surgeon*. Editor: Moshe Schein. tfm publishing Limited, 2003.

- *A Companion to Aphorisms & Quotations for the Surgeon*. Editor: Moshe Schein. tfm publishing Limited, 2008.

- *Schein's Common Sense Prevention and Management of Surgical Complications*. Editors: Schein, Rogers, Leppäniemi, Rosin. tfm publishing Limited, 2013.

- *Schein's Common Sense Emergency Abdominal Surgery,* 4th ed. Editors: Schein, Rogers, Leppäniemi, Rosin, Efron. tfm publishing Limited, 2015.

Artist's note

I've been doing surgery for about 20 years. I've been drawing cartoons for longer than that. At first they were just an outline of my 'surgical impressions'; later, gradually, I tried looking at surgery through the prism of humor. For even in the most serious situations there is always a place for jokes.

And now — we have a whole book. Even in my wildest dreams I could not imagine that would happen.

I cannot find words to express my gratitude and appreciation to the publisher, Nikki Bramhill from tfm publishing, the 'ideological catalyst' Moshe Schein, and my good friends Vyacheslav Ryndine and Denis Arkhipov.

Please direct comments, suggestions and opinions to perya70@gmail.com.

Evgeniy (Perya) Perelygin MD
Perm Clinical Center
Perm, Russia

Editor's note

Let me assure you that the humourless as a bunch don't just not know what's funny; they don't know what's serious. They have no common sense, either, and shouldn't be trusted with anything.

Martin Amis

Years ago I came across a few caricatures by a young surgeon from Siberia. His name was Evgeniy Perelygin — known to his friends as Perya. In a few black and white lines Perya managed to capture the funny, the amusing, and the ridiculous aspects of what we surgeons do or think. Yes, we surgeons take our profession very seriously and our patients even more seriously. But, what is true in any aspect of human life and endeavor is true for surgery — there is always something to laugh about, to paint in grotesque colors, or even to ridicule. And this includes, above all — ourselves.

Luckily, I managed to recruit Perya to 'decorate' a few of our surgical textbooks with his amazing caricatures. As is often the case, not everyone was appreciative of our mixing 'funny cartoons' and 'serious surgery'. A few surgeons who reviewed our books were appalled by the inclusion of "silly cartoons" amidst the "otherwise excellent chapters". I gather that for them anything to do with surgery is sacred — it was almost as if one had taken the holy Bible and decorated it with caricatures of Jesus.

But we are familiar with the types who avoid humor, do not understand jokes and enslave themselves to the steadily growing religion of political correctness which contaminates all our workplaces. We know who they are and the danger they pose to our humanity. Because humor, sarcasm, satire, criticism were always, and still are, the weapons of the smart and bright to resist the officious and dogmatic individuals who constantly wish to control our behavior.

The aim of this book is to introduce Perya's work to the international surgical community. I hope that some readers will use the images to enliven their boring PowerPoint lectures.

So stop taking yourself so seriously, do not be afraid to laugh or make others laugh. If anyone does not appreciate your humor… he/she can kiss your ass!

A life without a sense of humor has no sense at all.

Moshe Schein MD FACS
Marshfield Clinic, Ladysmith
Wisconsin, USA

P.S. I wish to thank Dr. Slava Ryndine for introducing Perya to me.

Thanks also to my friends Paul Rogers (for kindly proofing the whole manuscript and his wise advice), Ahmad Assalia, Ari Leppäniemi, Danny Rosin, and Jon Efron — my partners in the books in which many of the caricatures originally appeared. Many thanks also to the members of SURGINET for their interest and (often hilarious) advice.

The little book of surgical cartoons

1 The surgeon

Ideal life

Wishful thinking...

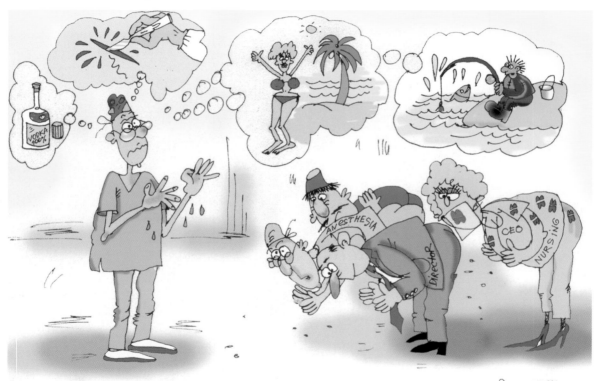

Surgeons are a little too apt to treat their art as an entrancing hobby, rather than an instrument capable of doing great good and unspeakable harm.

William Heneage Ogilvie, 1887-1971

Best surgeon in town

"WTF! I told them to bury only at night."

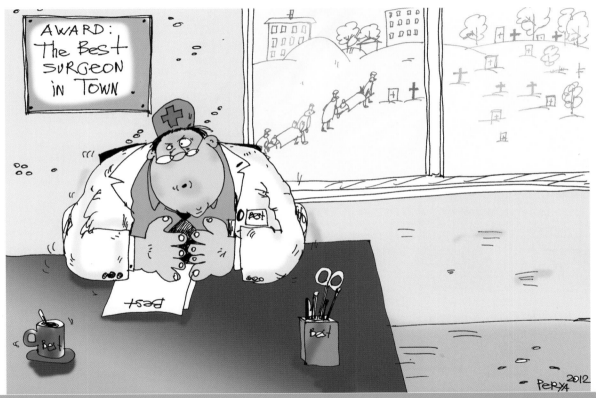

Every surgeon carries about him a little cemetery, in which from time to time he goes to pray, a cemetery of bitterness and regret, of which he seeks the reason for certain of his failures.

René Leriche, 1879-1955

The macho surgeon

"I'm a little tired... I did two 'Whipples' this morning."

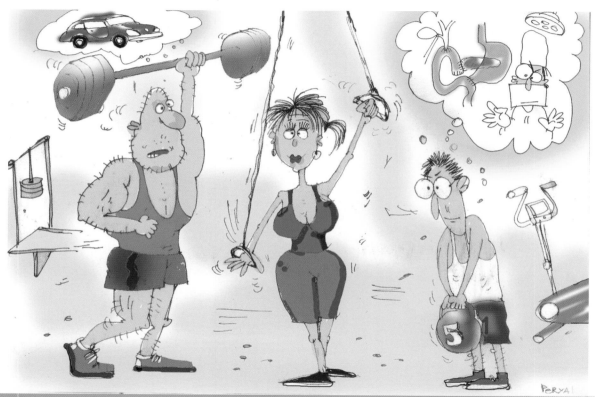

In ancient Greece they believed in hubris and nemesis. These concepts seem to resonate with surgery. If you are arrogant or boastful [hubris] about your surgery, the next case that you operate upon will go horribly wrong [nemesis].

David Dent

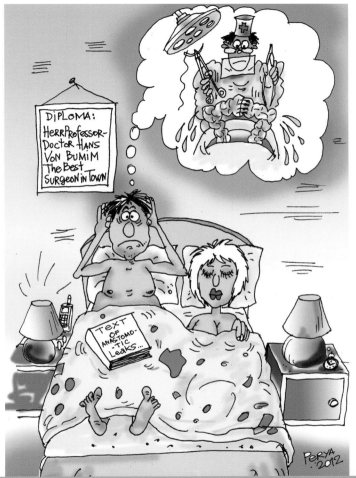

The worrying surgeon

Surgeon: "Will it leak? I should have added another layer."
Wife: "Take some valium!"

I have many colleagues, all of varying levels of knowledge and skill... But the ones I trust most are the ones that worry. You can see the concern, sometimes even anguish on their faces. Then, ... there are the sociopaths...

Tom Gilas

Scientific honesty

"This is my boss. We lost 5 cases before the study began. One died after the abstract had been submitted..."

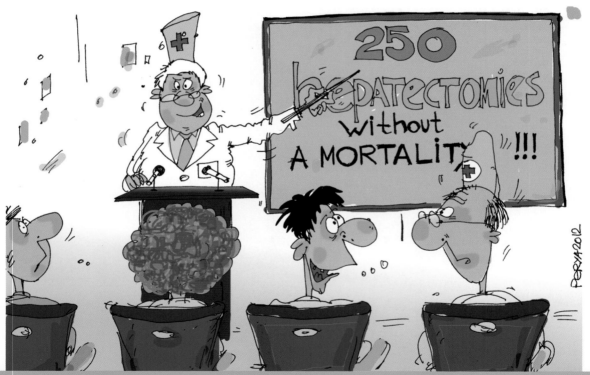

Scientific truth, which I formerly thought of as fixed, as though it could be weighted and measured, is changeable. Add a fact, change the outlook, and you have a new truth.

William J. Mayo, 1861-1939

The surgeon

Think like an infantry soldier going to combat!

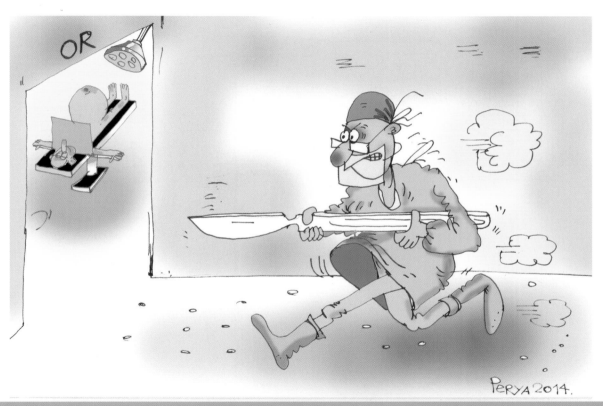

He who wishes to be a surgeon should go to war.

Hippocrates, 460-377 BC

Administrators vs. surgeons

Administrators:
"No patients, no surgeons, lots of money…"

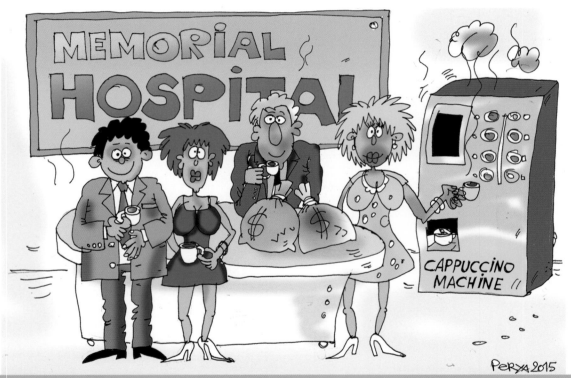

There is a growing gap in world view and usage of work-related lingo between hospital administrators and surgeons. It seems that the only term which still keeps them together is "$".

MS

Surgeons:
"Lots of money, many 'cases', no administrators…"

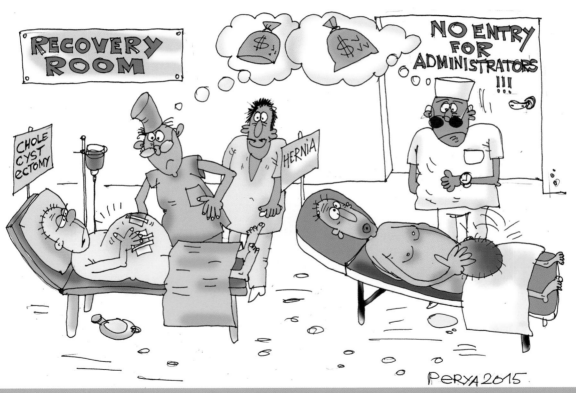

There are only four forms of incentive that I now, in my 27th year as a surgical chair, recognise: cash, money, cash money, and everything that can be converted into cash money.

Josef Fischer

The rural surgeon

"Doc, come back — you have a case!"

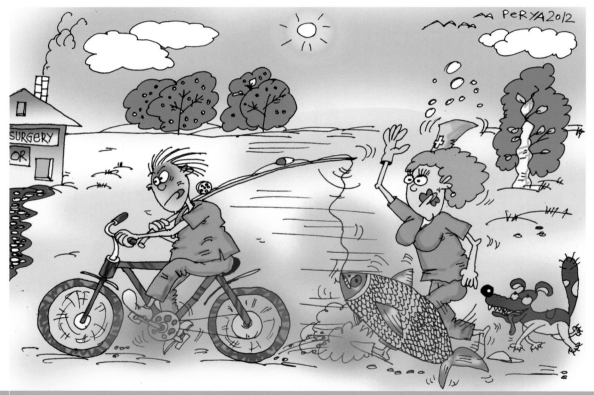

As long as the patient has an appendix, a gallbladder, a uterus and two ovaries, you refer them to the rural surgeon. Once these organs are gone you refer them to the city.

MS

The bariatric surgeon

"Doc, which procedure should we choose? I was offered a modelling contract pending a BMI of 22 within 3 months..."

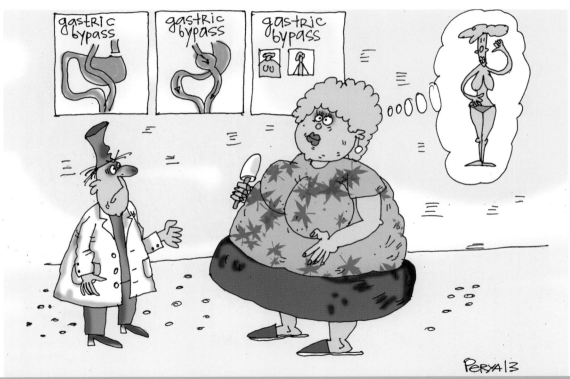

For the vast majority of patients today, there is no operation that will control weight to a 'normal' level without introducing risks and side effects that over a lifetime may raise questions about its use for surgical treatment of obesity.

Edward E. Mason

The breast surgeon

"Our mastectomy rate for breast cancer is zero! This is another fantastic cosmetic result of breast-conserving surgery!"

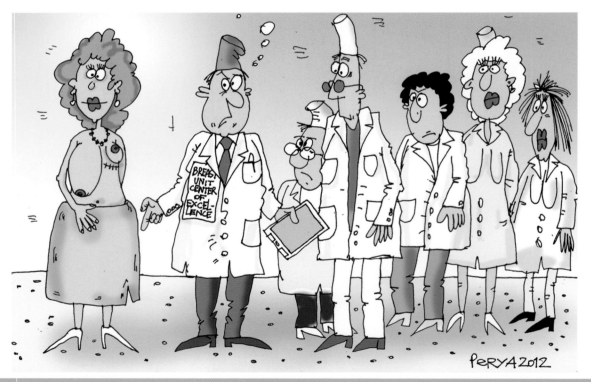

There is a huge 'breast industry' that feeds itself on the anxieties of breast cancer-prone women.

2 The practice

Gynecologists and the 'acute abdomen'

"Call the general surgeon... I think it is appendicitis..."

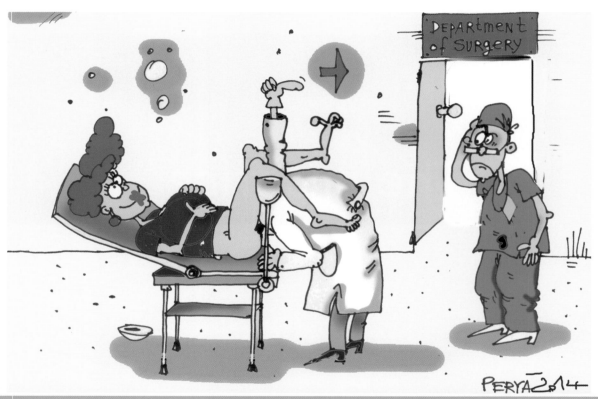

Have you ever seen a gynecologist who is convinced that the 'acute abdomen' is gynecological in origin, and not due to acute appendicitis?

MS

Check lists and wrong-side surgery

Defense lawyer: "It is not his fault. All check lists were OK."
Plaintiff's lawyer: "He should have re-examined her before the operation!"

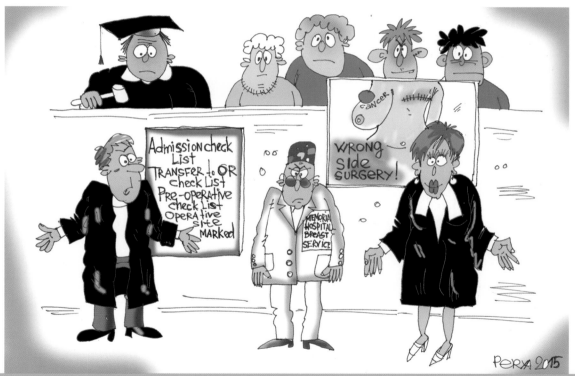

The nurses and OR staff will go over the check list de jour, mark the operative site and "time out" will be conducted but all such precautions are prone to human error. You have to conduct your own check list!

Rural hospitals vs. ivory towers

"A shithole... bunch of quacks..."

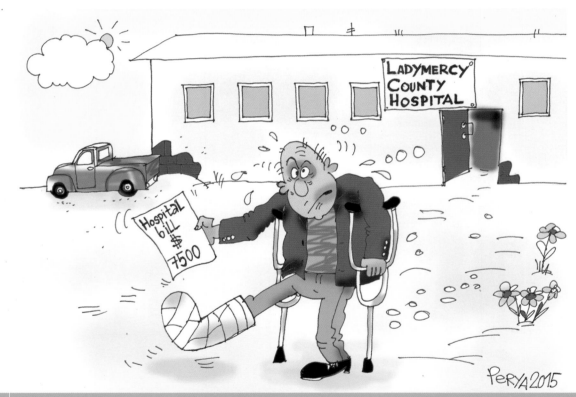

About managing acutely injured patients in U.S. rural hospitals: if you ship them away they'll accuse you of laziness, cowardice, or losing income for the hospital; but if you treat them locally they'll accuse you of being a 'cowboy' or endangering the patient.

"An excellent hospital — they saved my life!"

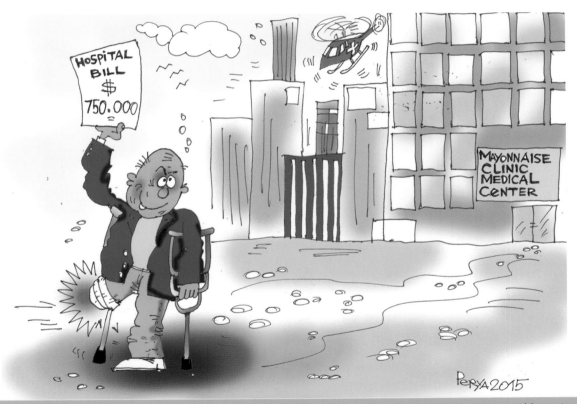

The common perception is that mortality or complications after an operation in a rural hospital are because of the "inexperienced surgeon or poor care" while if the patient dies in the Ivory Tower then he dies despite "the best efforts of the excellent doctors in a great hospital" — an act of God!

Anticoagulation

"Who takes aspirin, Plavix, Coumadin or Pradaxa?"

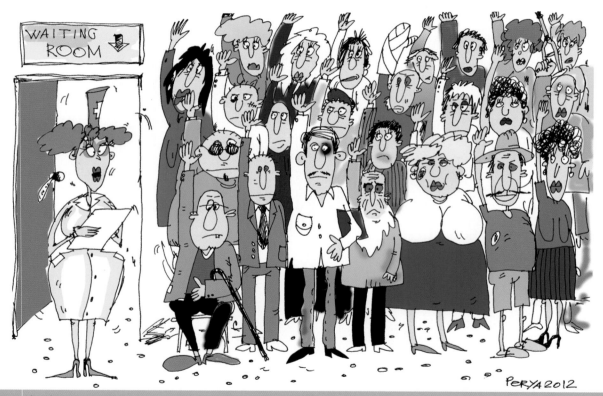

In today's surgical practice it is hard to find a patient who is not on any 'blood thinners'.

MS

Consultants

"Hey guys, where is Martha — the clinical psychologist?"

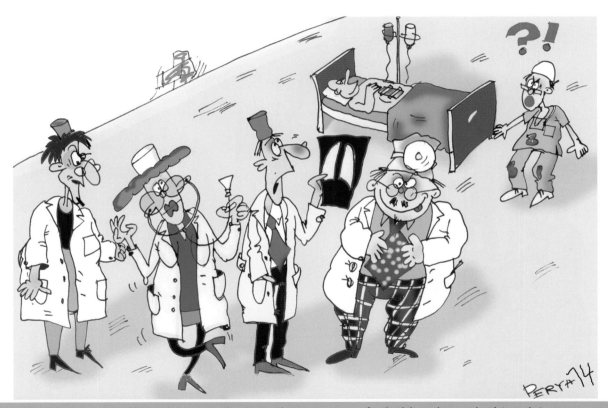

The problem with calling in a consultant is that you may feel obliged to take his advice.
Mark M. Ravitch, 1910-1989

The family

"Dear family, I am Dr. Mustafa, a general surgeon, and I am going to fix your husband and father..."

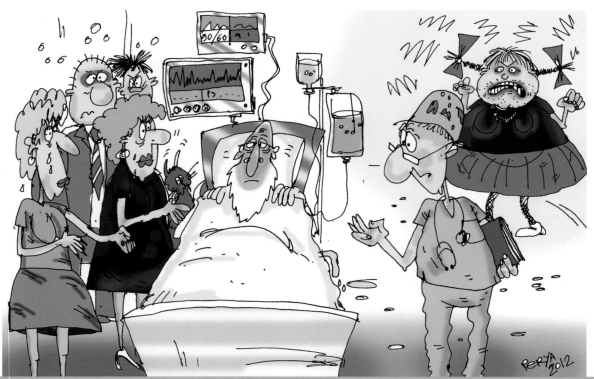

Risk management begins just when you first meet the patient and family. Acknowledge each member of the family — look into his or her eye — one of them (the one hiding in the corner) may be the one to initiate the lawsuit against you.

MS

Who is responsible?

"Who is responsible for this patient?"

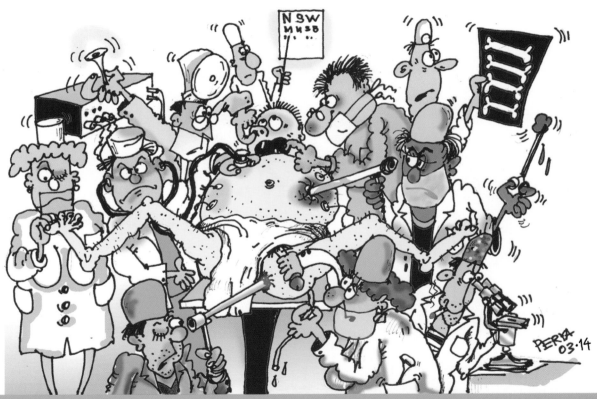

The surgeon may in some degree share his responsibilities with others, but the chief responsibility must always lie with him. And being his must be exercised not only during the operation but also before, perhaps long before, and also after, perhaps long after, the operation is performed.

Berkeley Moynihan, 1865-1936

21

The decision

The decision: Operate? Wait? Transfer?

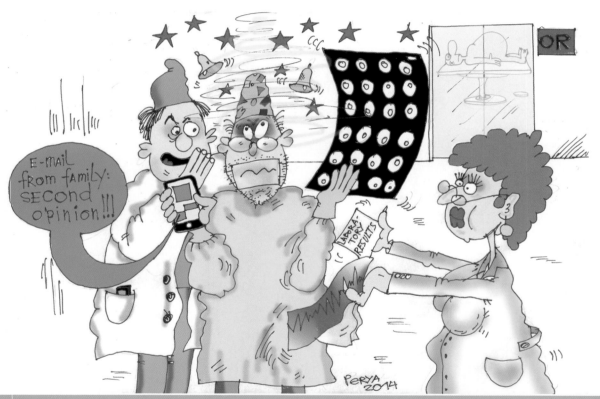

It is the surgeon himself who must take the final decision, and in making it he necessarily stands apart from his colleagues in a kind of loneliness.

Ian Aird, 1905-1962

Antibiotics

"Doc, try gorillacillin. It kills all bugs!"

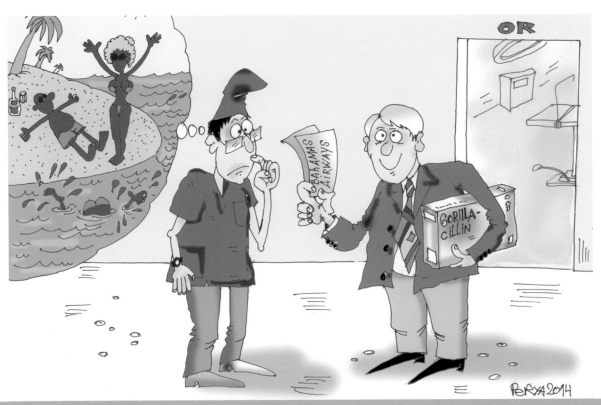

Patients can get well without antibiotics.

Mark M. Ravitch, 1910-1989

Informed consent

"Sir, please sign!"

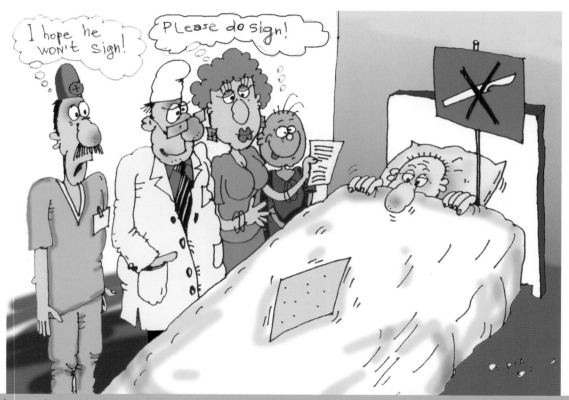

Informed consent is not the piece of paper, it is the process of understanding, and the agreement.
David Dent

Africa

"Wait, wait, I need a 2nd opinion!"

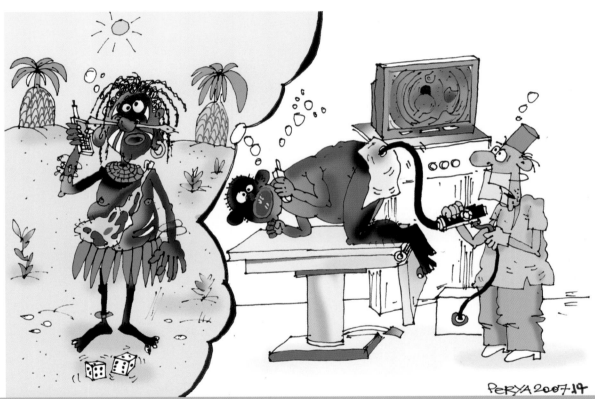

Anal electricity before urban electricity...   **Samir Johna**

They don't want the white man interfering with them; leave them to their own designs and let's see their prowess.

Johnny Dissidence (*Welcome to Hell: Experiences of White Doctors in Africa*)

Asia

Patient: "My ass is burning!"
Doctor: "Tell your wife to add more turmeric next time."

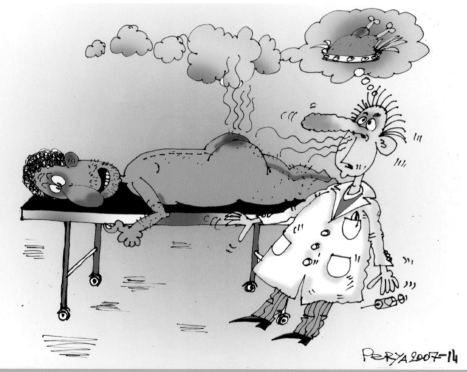

You must be aware of pathologies specific to the location.

Enhanced recovery after surgery (ERAS)

"Yes Sir, our cutting edge ERAS program is quite liberal…"

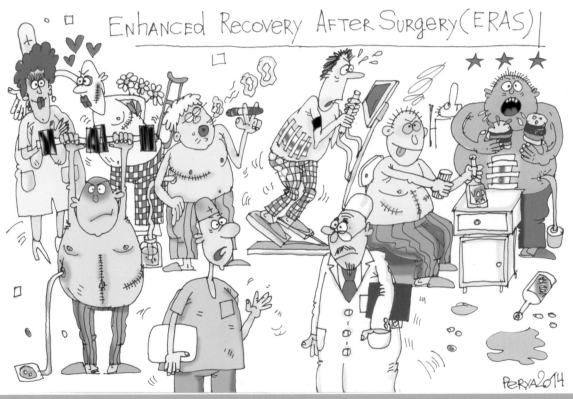

My rule of life prescribed as an absolutely sacred rite smoking cigars and also the drinking of alcohol before, after and if need be during all meals and in the intervals between them.

Winston Churchill, 1874–1965

Postoperative feeding

"Sir, she's a day after a total gastrectomy. I let them eat whatever they wish!"

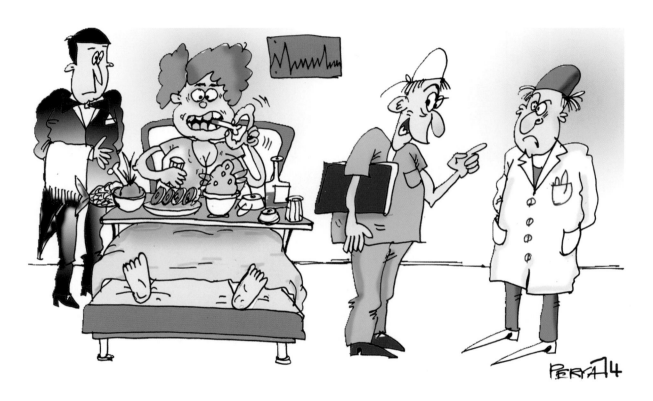

There is no way a patient is going to eat a hole in the anastomosis.

P. O. Nyström

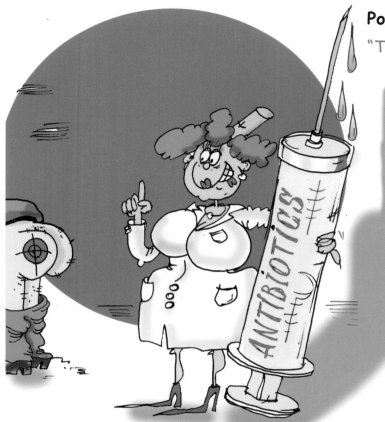

Postoperative antibiotics

"This will cure your SIRS..."

No amount of postoperative antibiotics can compensate for intra-operative mishaps and faulty technique, or can abort postoperative suppuration necessitating drainage.

Money matters

"Yes, a hopeless case... but we can still bill for it!"

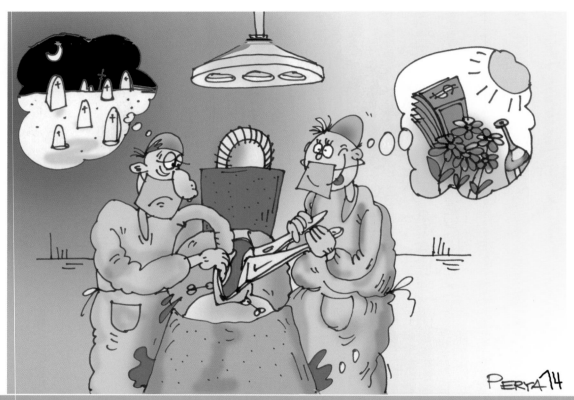

Unfortunately, the practice of surgery today is as much a business as it is a science and art.
Thomas R. Russell, 1940-2014

The Third World

Surgeon: "I can repair your hernia with a mosquito net. It will cost you 10 shillings."
Patient: "Can't you use a bioprosthesis?"

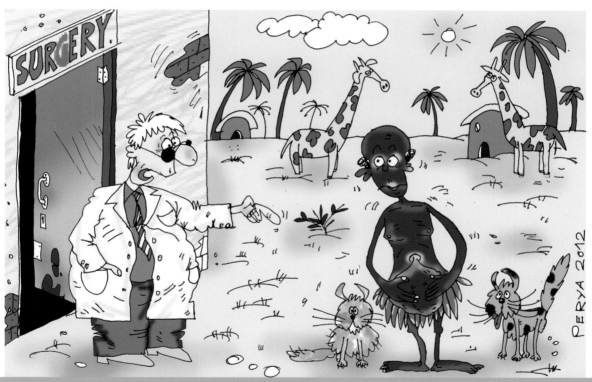

On Saturday, I was a surgeon in South Africa, very little known.
On Monday, I was world renowned.

Christiaan Barnard, 1922-2001

3 Modern days

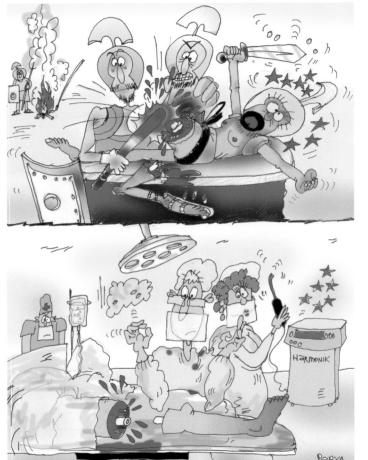

Surgical history

500 BC — "Perfect hemostasis! Now we can grill…"

2015 — "There is nothing like the harmonic scalpel!"

Same results!

Surgeons vs. pilots

"Doctor, show me your pilot license and CME certificates!"

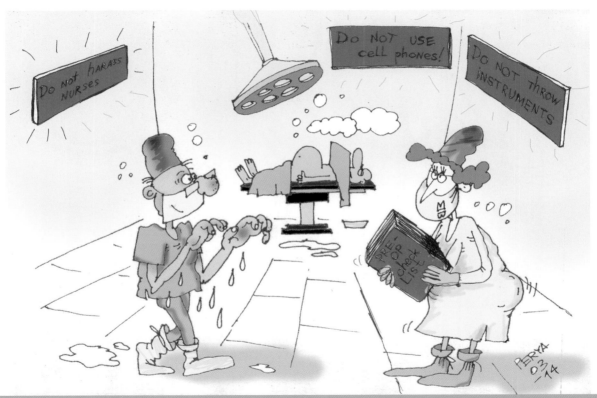

Pilots don't fill out a form documenting that they put a landing gear down. This is another fundamental difference in the two professions. We (surgeons) obsess about documentation; aviation worries about getting the wheels down.

Richard C. Karl

35

Minimally invasive surgery

Old fart: "Minimally invasive appendectomy, really...?"

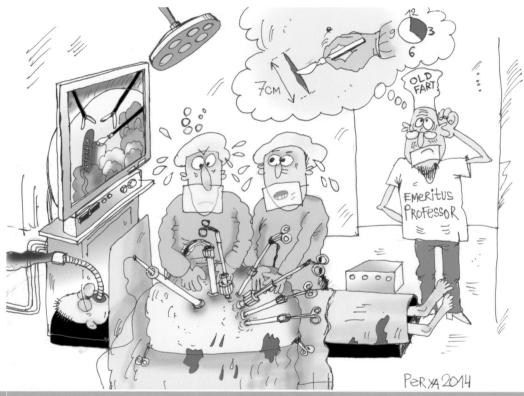

I know lots of anaesthetists who rely upon anecdote to judge us surgeons. Almost to a man (or a woman) they regard laparoscopic surgery as a means by which straightforward operations that used to be done quickly now take hours and inevitably involve vast quantities of disposable kit.

John MacFie

The learning curve

Scrub nurse: "Doc, should we cancel the last two cases?"
Surgeon: "Shhhh. Let me reach the top of the learning curve!"

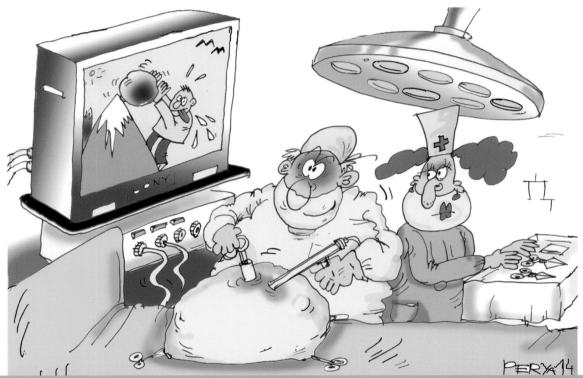

This procedure has a long learning curve; you have to screw up a large number of unsuspecting patients before you can master it.

Kuldip Pandey

Single-incision laparoscopic surgery

"Looks lovely! A beautiful wound! I told you that my single-incision lap surgery is the way to go..."

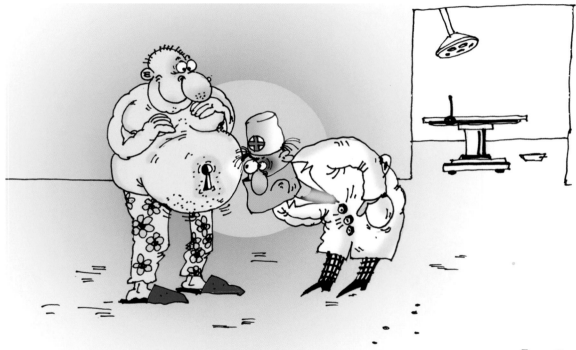

SILS (single-incision laparoscopic surgery) is SILLY.

Mark Cheetham

Natural orifice transluminal endoscopic surgery

Assistant: "Should we remove the lipoma with NOTES?"
Surgeon: "NOTES (natural orifice transluminal endoscopic surgery) is NUTS!"

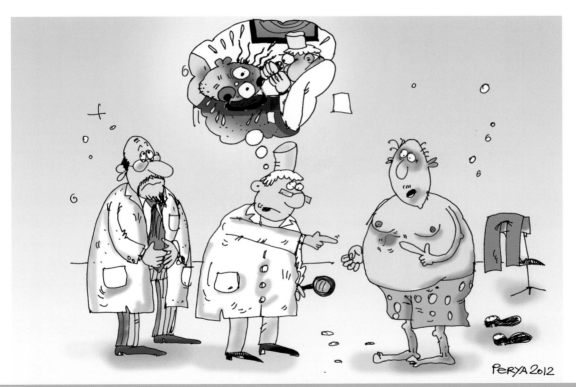

A rule of thumb is that the tumor should be removed by laparotomy and not laparoscopy if it is bigger than the head of the surgeon in question.

David Dent

39

Robotic surgery

Surgeon: "WTF is that?"
Resident: "Sir, the CEO wants us to utilize the new robot..."

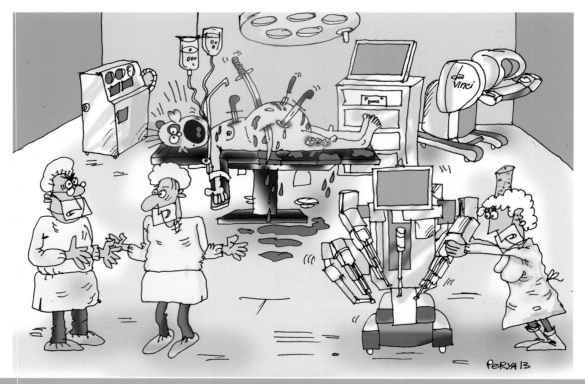

If you can't do it with the laparoscope alone, you shouldn't do it with the robot.
If you can do it with the laparoscope, you don't need the robot.

Mark Pleatman

Computed tomography

"But I had a CT last year!"

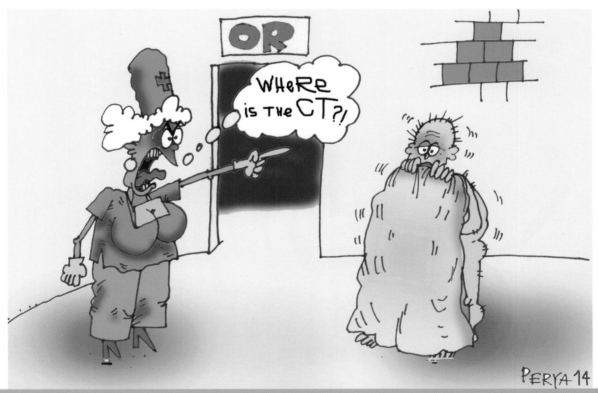

Luckily, gone are the days when the acute abdomen represented a totally black box. In the individual patient it helps us to be more selective and more conservative, and to decide when not to operate and when to choose alternative modalities...

MS

Up-to-date generation

"What about examining the patient? Is this mentioned on your i-phone?"

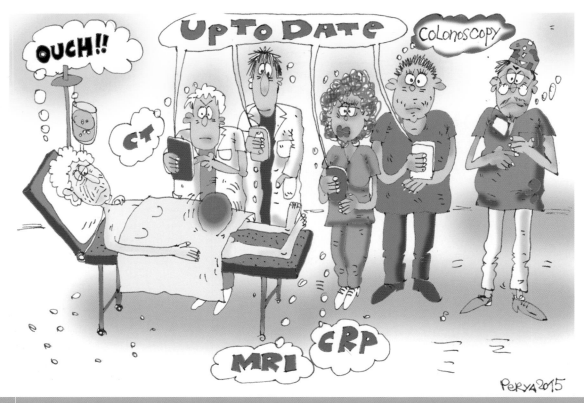

The examining physician often hesitates to make the necessary examination because it involves soiling his finger.

William J. Mayo, 1861-1939

Shift mentality

Surgeon: "Where are you going guys? He's bleeding to death!"
Residents: "We are going home. Our shift has finished..."

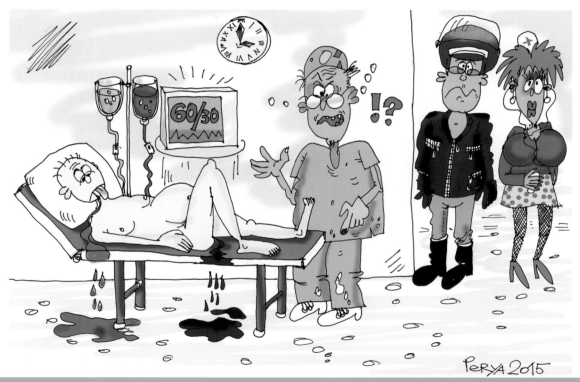

Shi(f)t happens...

Anestis Karakatsanis

Convert to laparoscopy

"Nurse, I'm lost. This operation is now beyond my scope. I need to close the abdomen and convert to laparoscopy!"

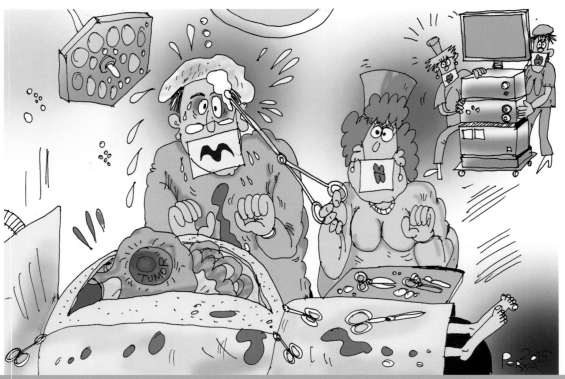

Let's face it, modern laparoscopic training has placed open surgery beyond the scope of many trainees.

Stephen Clifforth

Modern surgery in the Third World

An Indian to his friend: "Finally, modern medicine has arrived in Mumbai…"
The friend: "Do you think they would remove my hemorrhoids with the robot?
I have 3 dollars…"

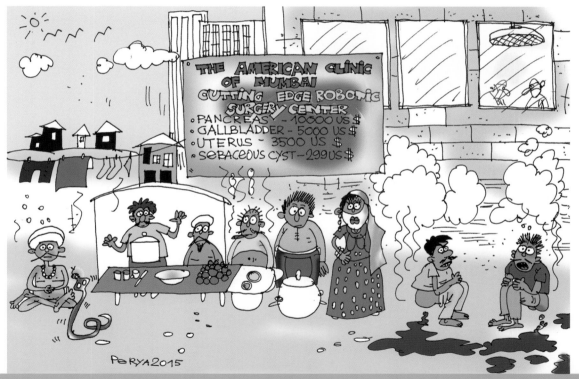

When technology is the Master, the result is Disaster!

We, the surgeons, are the most gimmick-conscious group of suckers of any other professionals in the world.

Eric Frykberg, 1951-2013

A modern residency program

Chief of Surgery to his residents — then...
"Who of you is good enough to assist me in a hernia?"

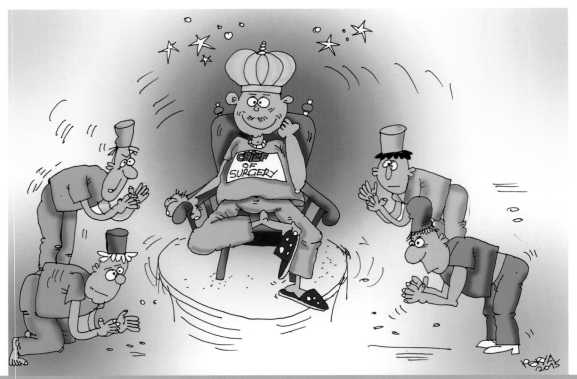

Resident involvement in an operation is earned. It must be clarified and delineated before the procedure begins.

Leo A. Gordon

and now...
"Please, please, would any of you let me assist you in a Whipple?"

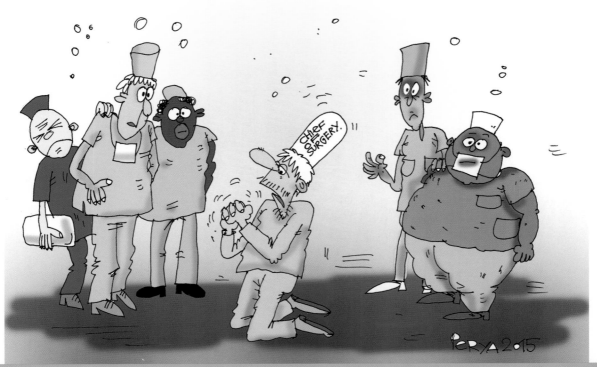

A good assistant does not always make a good chief, but a bad assistant never does. A good chief has always been a good assistant.

Charles F. M. Saint, 1886-1973

Modern 'non-profit' hospitals

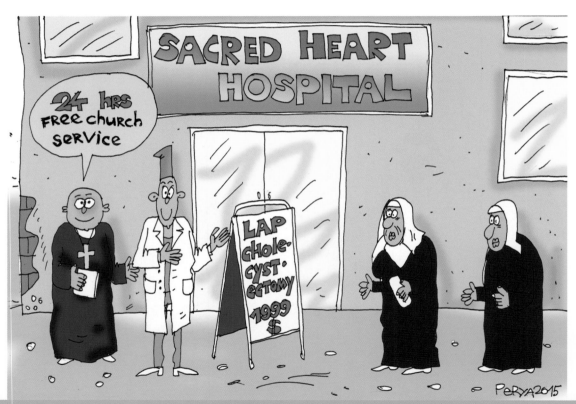

One of the things about the U.S. health care system is that it defies the laws of economics, and of gravity. Once the price is high, it just stays there...

Naoki Ikegami

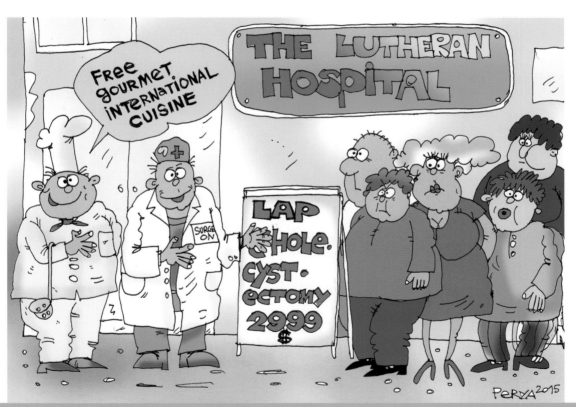

Know just this; a remuneration worthy of your labors, that is to say, a very good fee, makes for the authority of the physician and increases the confidence which the patient has in him, even if the physician be of great ignorance.

William of Salicet, 1210-1277

49

Modern 'non-profit' hospitals *continued*

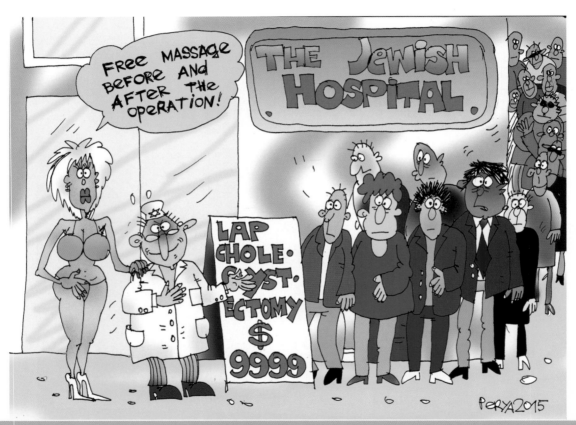

Commercialism and professionalism are parallel streams in our society that can coexist in peace. When they start to get mixed with each other, beware.

Francis D. Moore, 1913-2001

Cutting edge hospitals

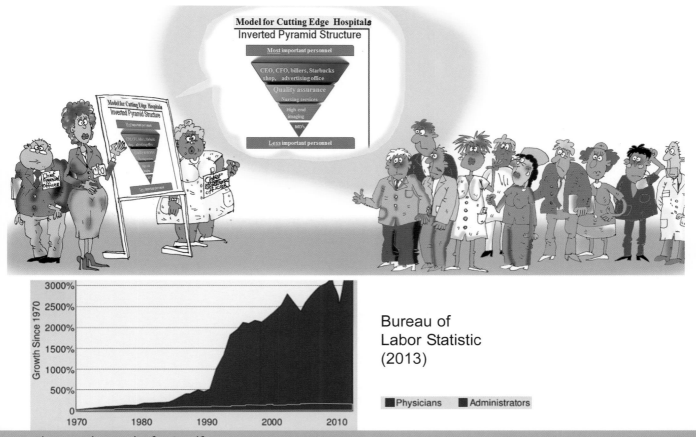

Bureau of
Labor Statistic
(2013)

The graph speaks for itself.

4 The abdomen

Penetrating abdominal trauma

"This is a classical case for non-operative management!"

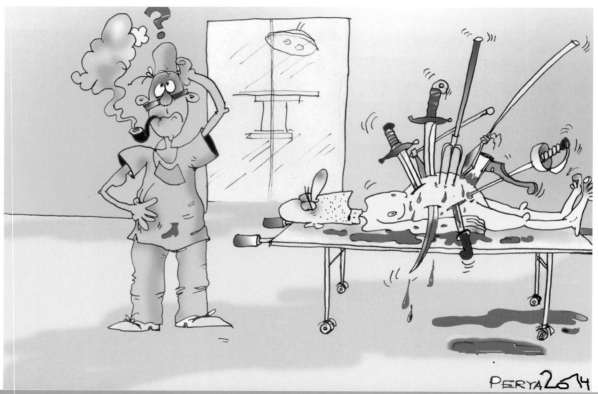

Failure to promptly recognize and treat simple life-threatening injuries is the tragedy of trauma, not the inability to handle the catastrophic or complicated injury.

F. William Blaisdell

Blunt abdominal trauma

"Doc, I think I need a CT!"

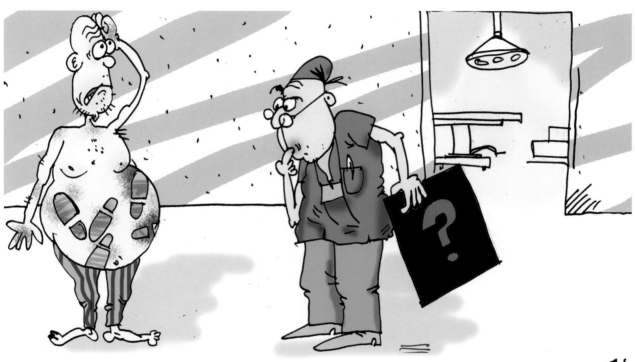

You cannot operate on a differential diagnosis.

Claude Organ, Jr., 1926-2005

Priorities in abdominal trauma

Surgeon: "I guess we have to stop the bleeding first!"
Assistant: "Sir, first let's deal with the contamination..."
Nurse: "Stop! Take him back to the ICU! According to the guidelines you have to rewarm him first."

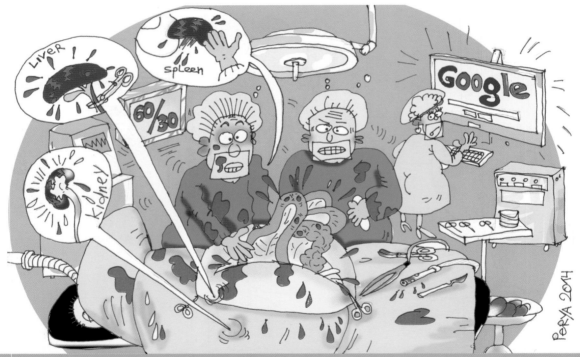

Know what you will do in the event you don't know what to do.

Rick Paul

The supreme surgeon uses his supreme judgment to avoid situations that would test his supreme abilities.

Pancreatic injury

"Doc, could I have a bite as well?"

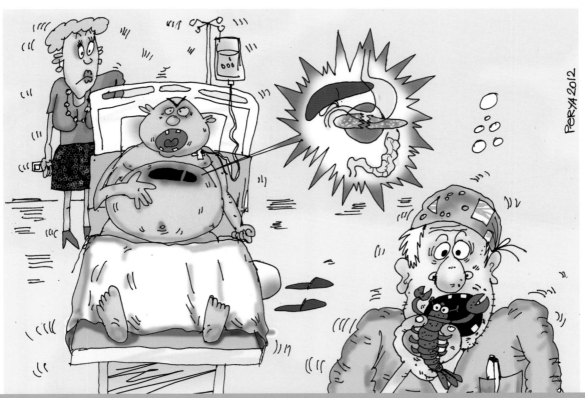

For pancreatic trauma: treat the pancreas like a crayfish, suck the head... eat the tail.
Timothy C. Fabian

Peritoneal lavage

"OK guys, I think it is enough, the abdomen is clean!"

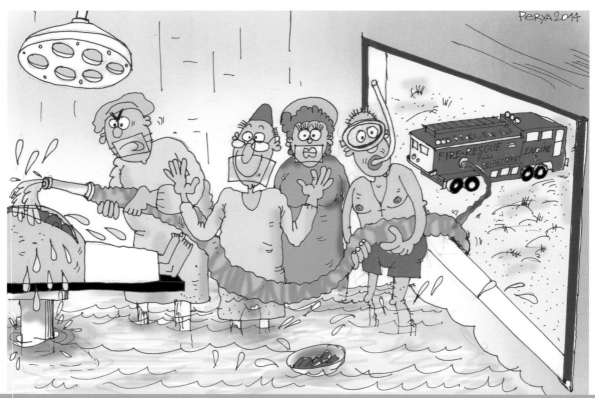

People claim that lavage is the solution to pollution by dilution of the contaminants — but remember that macrophages do not swim well.

MS

Acute abdomen

"Which of them has an 'acute abdomen'?"

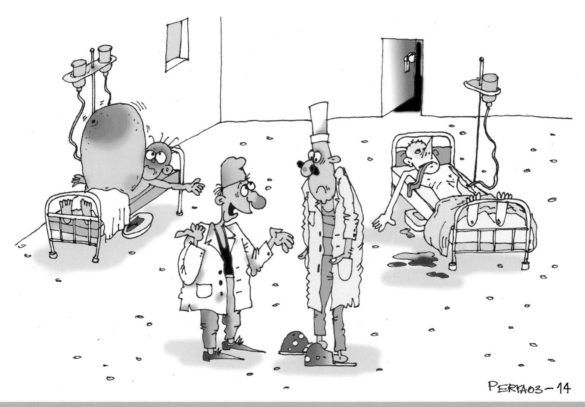

It is as much an intellectual exercise to tackle the problems of belly ache as to work on the human genome.

Hugh Dudley

Abdominal drains

"Which one is draining?"

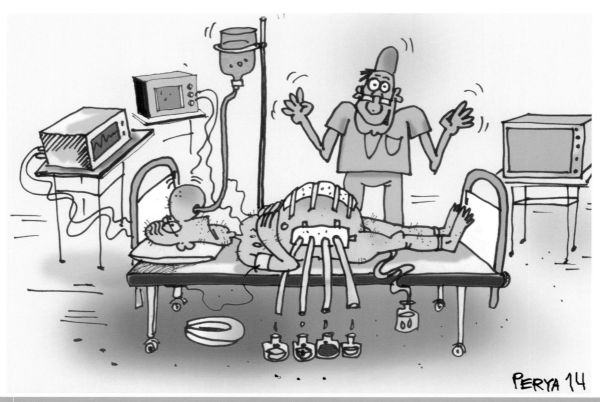

Drainage of the general peritoneal cavity is a physical and physiological impossibility.

J. L. Yates, ~1905

The best anastomosis

"My anastomosis is the best!"

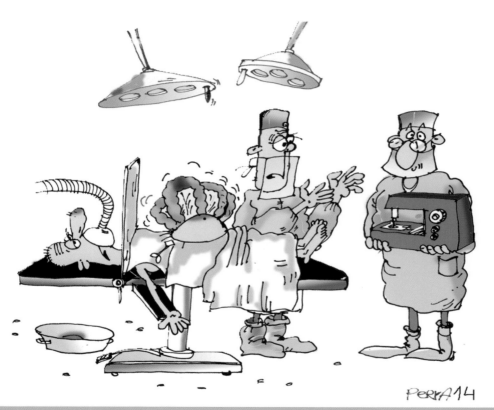

Anastomotic leakage is a completely avoidable complication — providing you don't perform an anastomosis.

Brendan Moran

Anastomosis vs. colostomy

"Should I anastomose? A colostomy?"

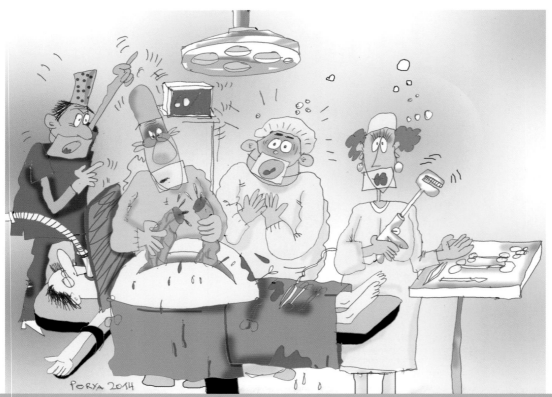

If you do a colostomy there will be always someone to ask "why not primary anastomosis?"
If you do a primary anastomosis there will be always someone to tell you "why not colostomy?"

MS

Colostomy in the kitchen?

"Nice colostomy, eh?"

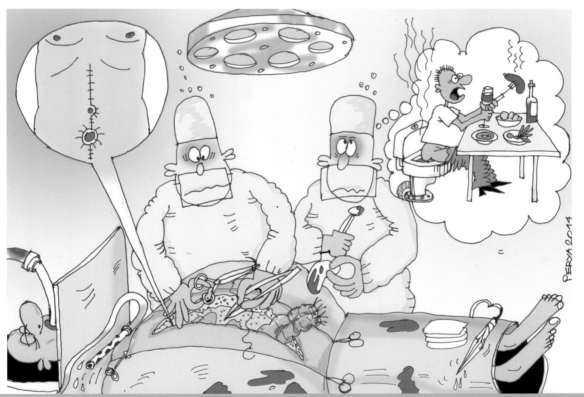

Bringing a colostomy out through a laparotomy incision is like putting a toilet in the kitchen…

Abdominal closure

"Pull harder! We have to prevent a hernia!"

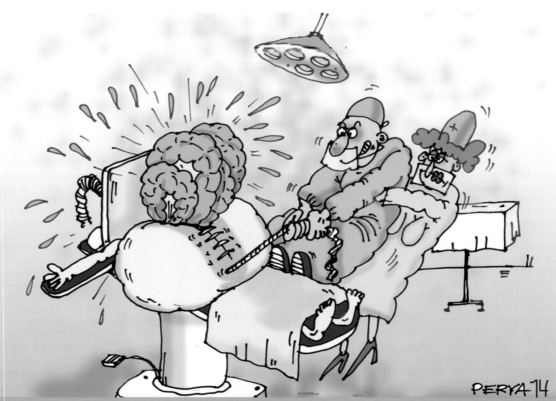

Abdominal closure: if it looks all right, it's too tight — if it looks too loose, it's all right.

Matt Oliver

Intra-abdominal hypertension

"He's huge! I am trying to prevent abdominal wall dehiscence!"

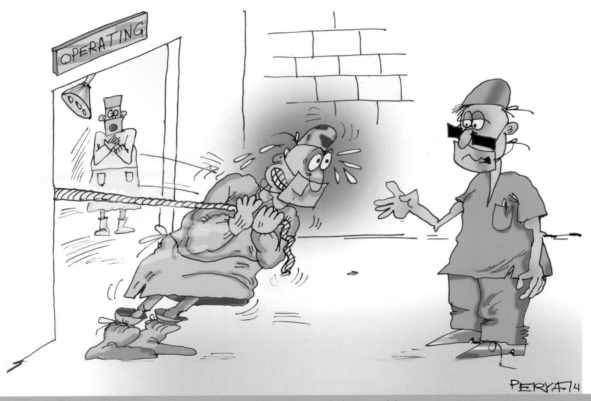

Abdominal closure under tension will produce intra-abdominal hypertension.

MS

Paraesophageal hernia

"Can I get a few more TUMS please...?"

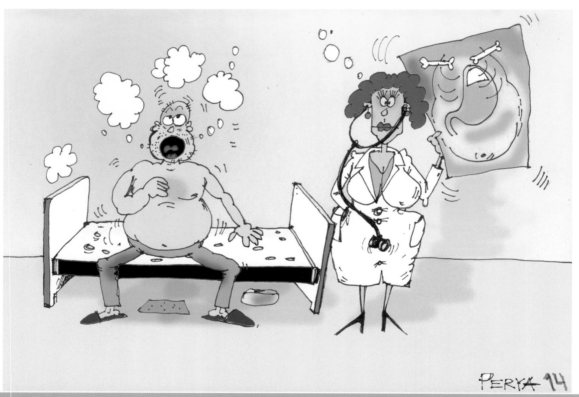

The diagnostic triad: epigastric/substernal pain, belching without vomiting, and the inability to pass a nasogastric tube.

Moritz Borchardt, 1868-1948

Upper gastrointestinal bleeding

"I think it is UGI bleeding!"

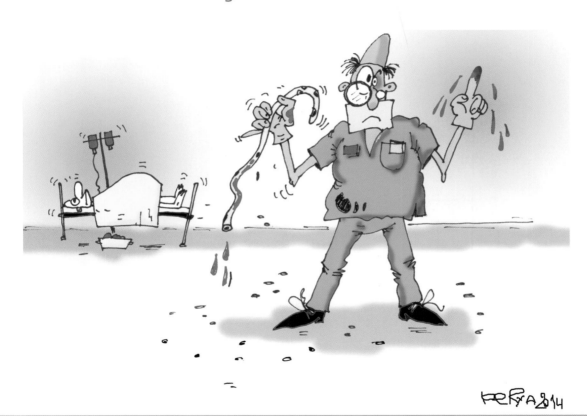

When the blood is fresh and pink and the patient is old, it is time to be active and bold.
When the patient is young and the blood is dark and old, you can relax and put your knife on hold.

MS

Perforated peptic ulcer

"How should I mend it? With a Graham patch?"

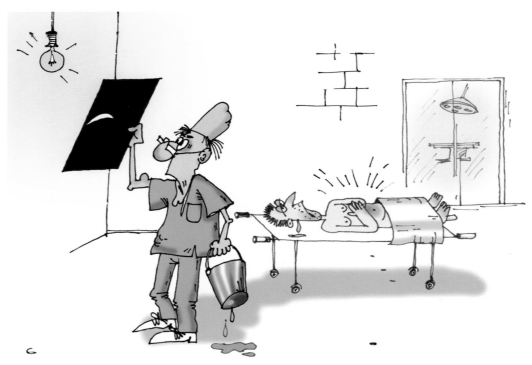

We have no responsibility to such patients but to save their lives. Any procedure, which aims to do more than this, can quite significantly be considered meddlesome surgery. We have no responsibility during the surgery to carry out any procedure to cure the patient of his duodenal ulcer.

Roscoe R. Graham, 1890-1948

Pancreatic necrosis

Assistant: "Prof, his pancreas is dead! When are we going to operate?"
Professor: "Patience! We'll operate, perhaps, next month. Now get me some more vino!"

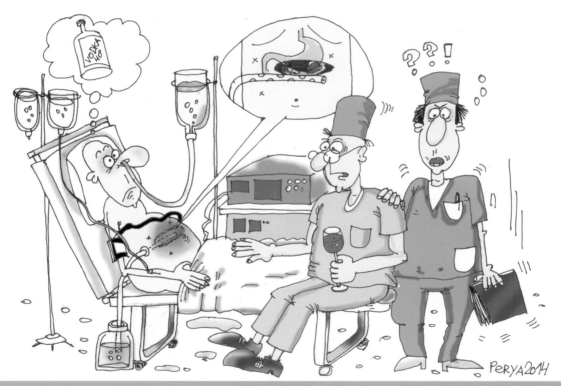

Acute pancreatitis is the most terrible of all the calamities that occur in connection with the abdominal viscera.

Berkeley Moynihan, 1865-1936

Biliary pancreatitis

"We found it!"

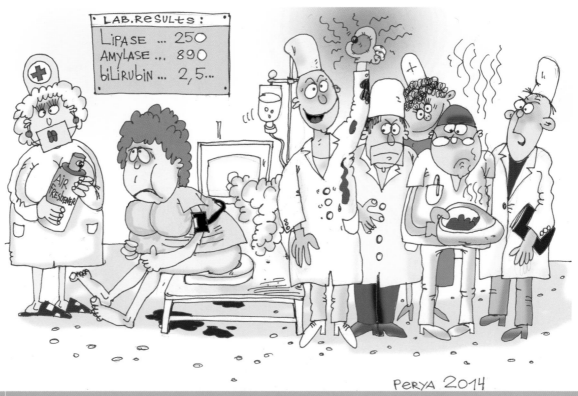

Gallstones are found in the feces of 34 out of 36 patients with pancreatitis.

Juan Miguel Acosta

Small bowel obstruction

"Is it ileus or obstruction? Let's try some Gastrografin®..."

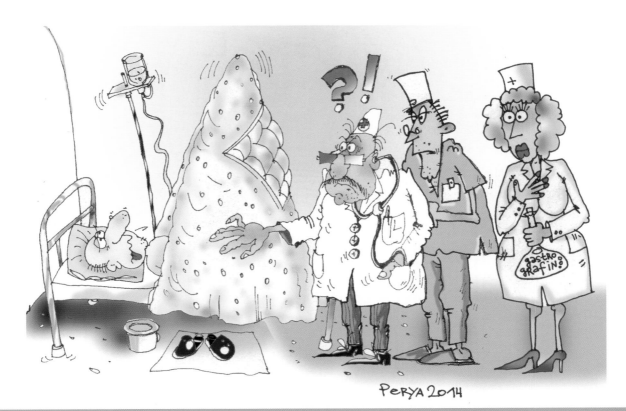

The only thing predictable about small bowel obstruction is its unpredictability.

MS

Laparoscopy in intestinal obstruction

"Let me try the laparoscope..."

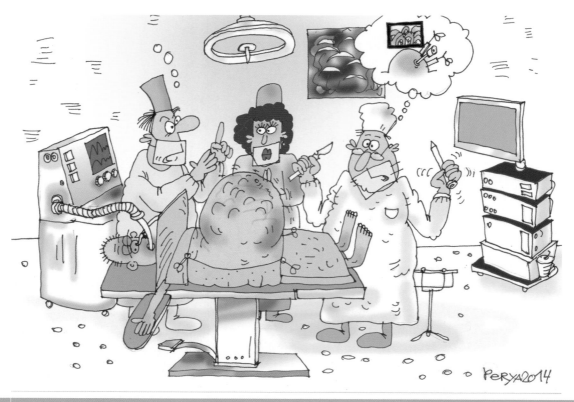

If you are too fond of new remedies, first you will not cure your patients; secondly, you will have no patients to cure.

Astley Paston Cooper, 1768-1841

Acute appendicitis

"It is not your tooth — it is your appendix!"

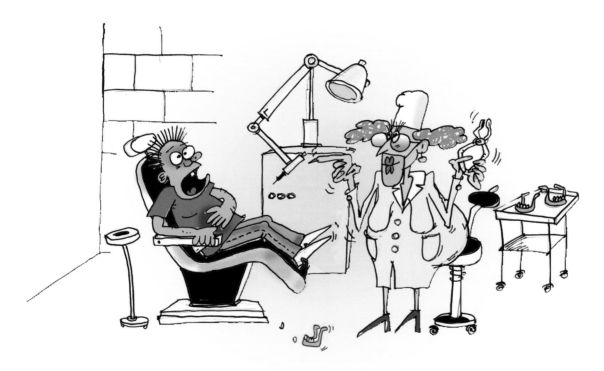

Even a dentist can diagnose classical acute appendicitis.

MS

Acute mesenteric ischemia

"How much should I resect?"

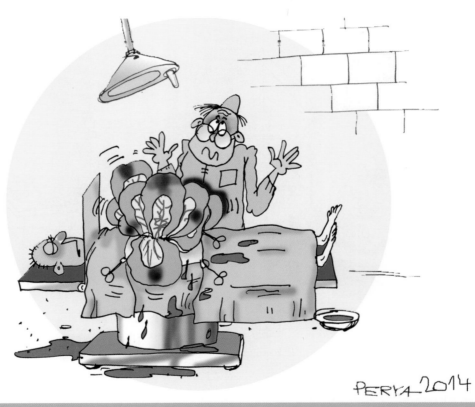

Occlusion of the mesenteric vessels is regarded as one of those conditions of which the diagnosis is impossible, the prognosis hopeless, and the treatment almost useless.

A. Cokkinis, ~1921

Ulcerative colitis

"You have pancolitis. You are toxic! No need for an operation... I am going to increase the Imuran..."

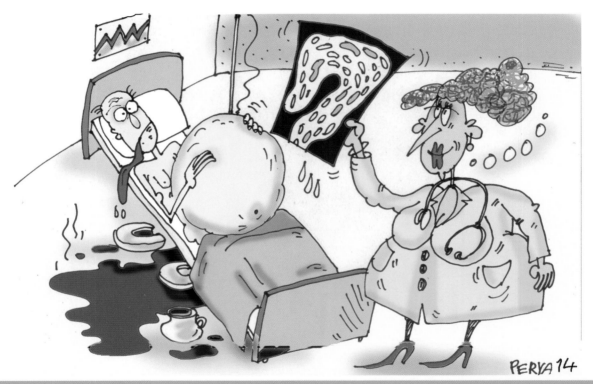

The simple wisdom is that failure of medical treatment should be recognized early — being an indication for surgical treatment. The worse the previous course has been — the stronger the indication for a colectomy during the current attack.

P. O. Nyström

Clostridium difficile colitis

Surgeon: "Anyone ready to serve as a shit donor for this poor *C. diff* patient?"
Medical student of the year: "Sir, what about an autotransplant?"

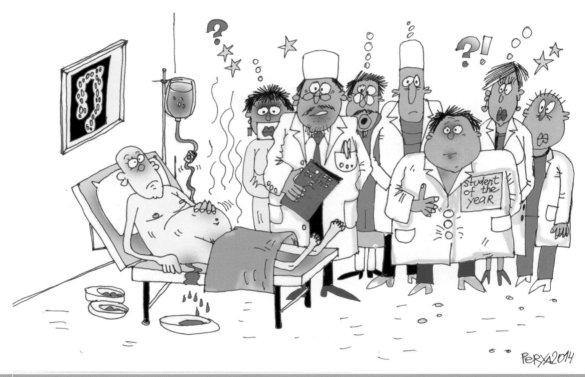

Fecal transplant... finally there's some BS that works.

John Kennedy

Sigmoid volvulus

"I can cure his volvulus without an operation!"

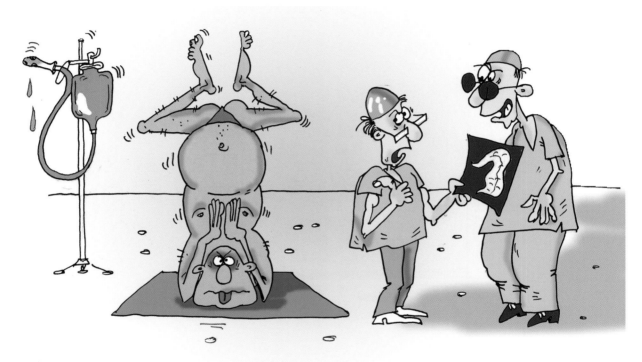

A rigid proctoscope made in 1935, when properly used to detort a sigmoid volvulus, can do more than any GI fellow with a $50,000 model x-6700 three-chip video laser-CD-ROM triply-enhanced surround-sound colonoscope.

Leo A. Gordon

Acute diverticulitis

"Hey, show me the one which is inflamed, so we know what to remove."

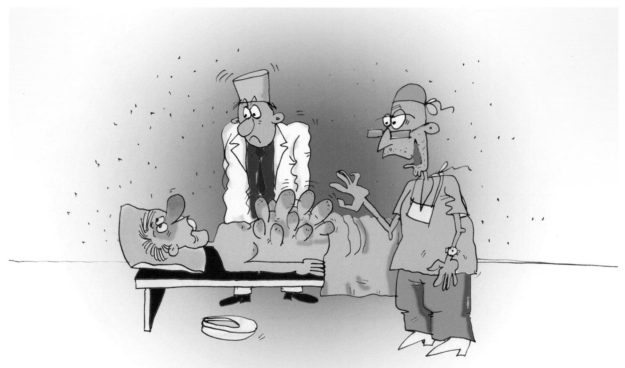

It is greatly more to the surgeon's credit to avoid, than to perform an operation – to arrest the progress of pathology instead of operating to remove it.

Max Thorek, 1880-1960

Perforated sigmoid diverticulitis

Medical student: "Sir, why didn't you get a CT? This would have responded to antibiotics…"

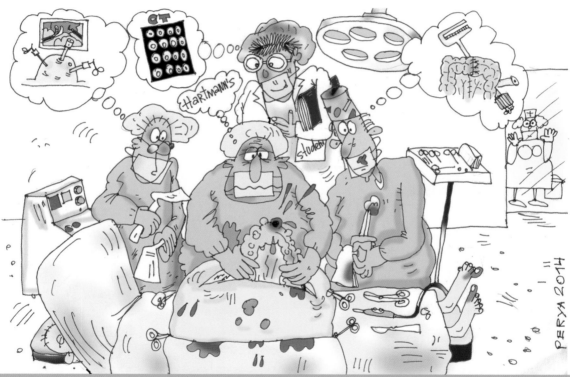

Intuition is the fastest way to reach a wrong solution.

Dick van Geldere

Lower gastrointestinal bleeding

"Boss, isn't this UGI bleeding? Want me to pass a nasogastric tube?"

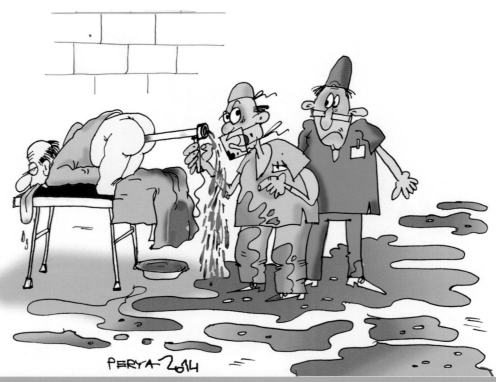

All bleeding eventually ceases.

Guy de Chauliac, 1300-1368

Abdominal compartment syndrome

Consultant: "Aren't you going to decompress them?"
Surgeon: "No Sir, we are waiting for them to eviscerate…"

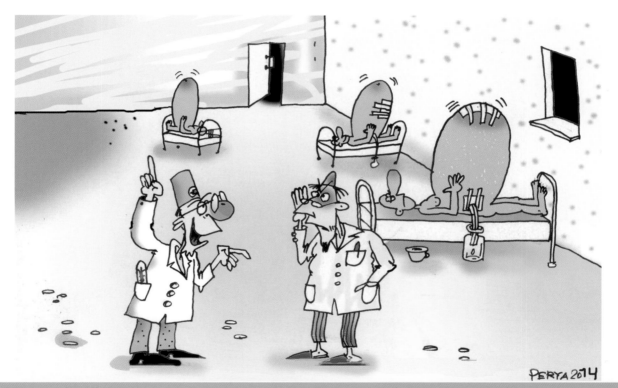

Abdominal wall dehiscence is how the patient treats his own abdominal compartment syndrome.

MS

Abdominal drainage

Surgical resident: "Sir, he's still spiking high temperatures…"
Infectious disease consultant: "I would insert a few more drains under CT!"

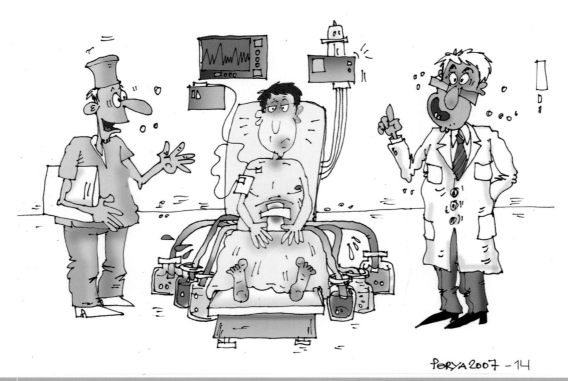

That you call something a drain does not guarantee that it actually drains.

Rick Paul

Before closing the abdomen...

Surgeon: "Should I leave him open? Close him up?"
Anesthetist: "How long will it take him to decide...?"

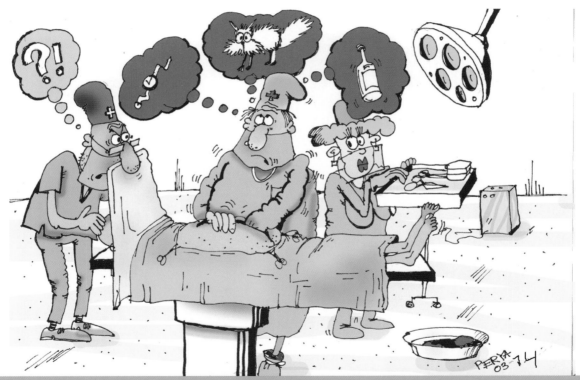

Do not compromise. Keep looking around; there's always something you've missed. Remember: when the abdomen is open you control it, when closed it controls you!

Postoperative ileus

Nurse: "Doctor, is this paralytic ileus?"
Doctor: "Shhhh, let me listen. I hear a single bowel sound — this must be mechanical obstruction."

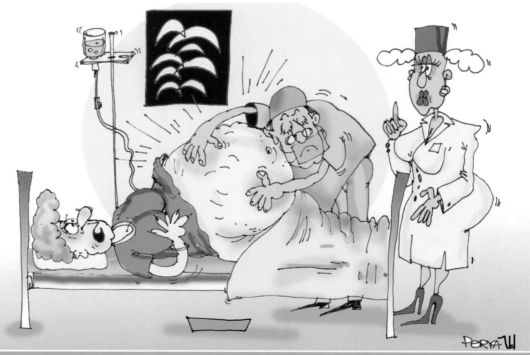

The truth is that in most instances the patient will improve spontaneously without you ever knowing whether it was an early postop mechanical small bowel obstruction or just an ileus.

MS

Abdominal auscultation

Intern: "Hurray! I hear some farting!"
Nurse: "Can't be, I do not hear any peristalsis whatsoever…"

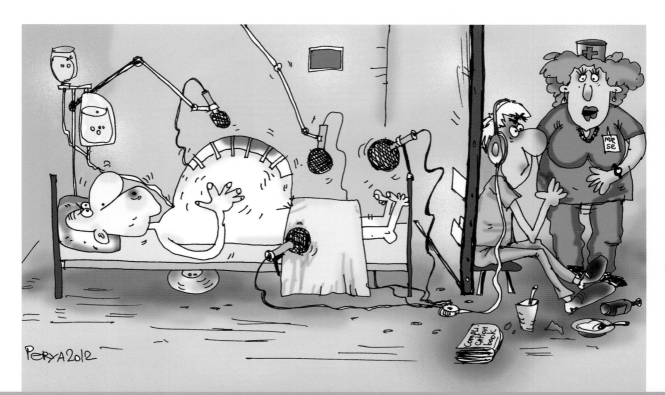

The postoperative fart is the best music to the surgeon's ears.

MS

Abdominal re-exploration

Junior: "Should I re-explore him?"
Senior: "Well, it all depends on his level of CRP... well, let me call my wife..."

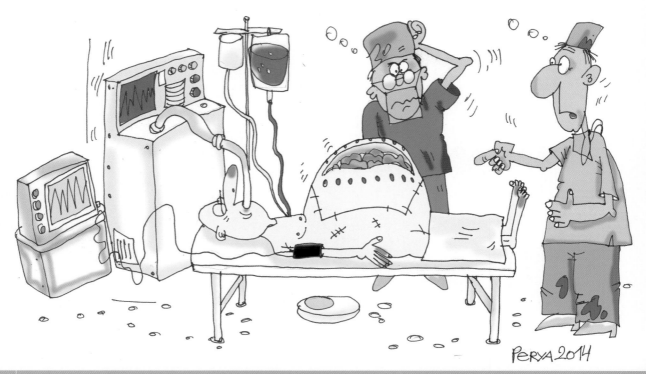

Frequent dilemma: take your spouse for dinner or the patient back to the OR? You may lose even if you make the correct choice.

Laparostomy

"We leave the abdomen open to let out the molecules of systemic and local inflammatory response syndrome..."

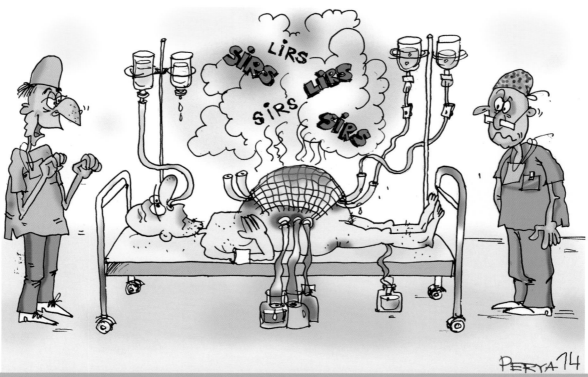

Consider laparostomy either when the abdomen cannot be closed or should not be closed.

Temporary abdominal closure

"This is our new temporary abdominal closure device. We believe in applying a vacuum to the whole patient!"

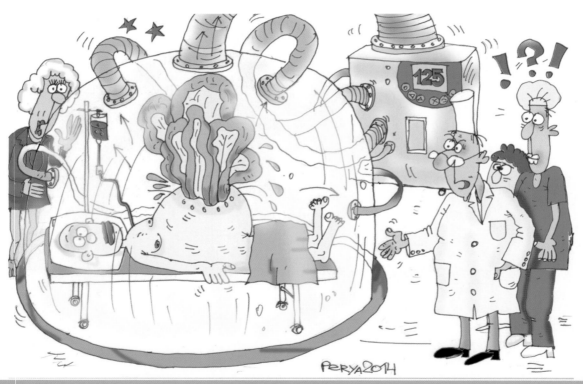

It usually requires a considerable time to determine with certainty the virtues of a new method of treatment and usually still longer to ascertain the harmful effects.

Alfred Blalock, 1899-1964

The abdominal incision

"Nurse, which incision?"

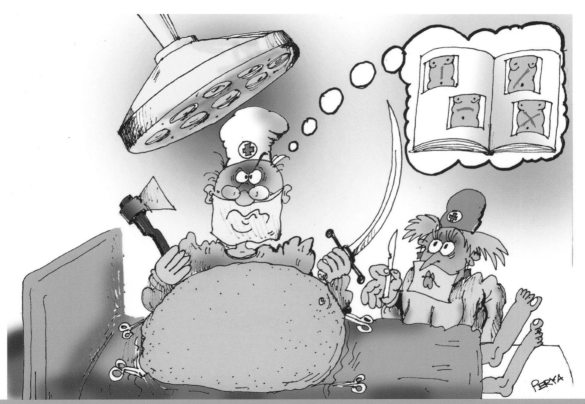

When the doctor is in doubt and the patient in danger, make an exploratory incision and deal with what you find as best as you can.

Robert Lawson Tait, 1845-1899

Abdominal exposure

"Hey Doc, why don't you extend it a little?"

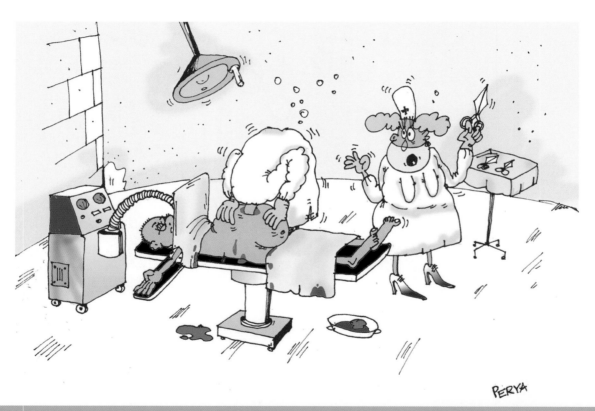

Surgery like lovemaking must be done gently and with adequate exposure.

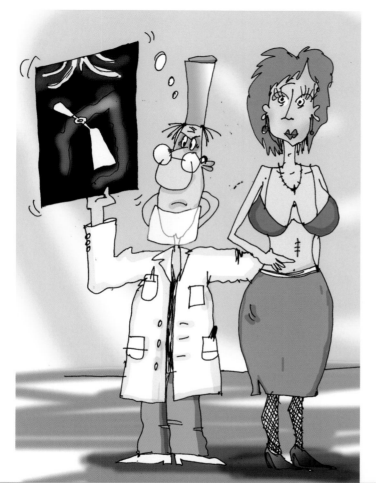

The abdominal wound

"Doctor, I am so happy: the scar is so little — I will be able to wear the bikini!"

The surgical wound is the only remnant of your operation the patient can actually see.

MS

5 Complications

Scrotal eggplant after hernia repair

"Doc, and you promised that I could go to Disneyland next week..."

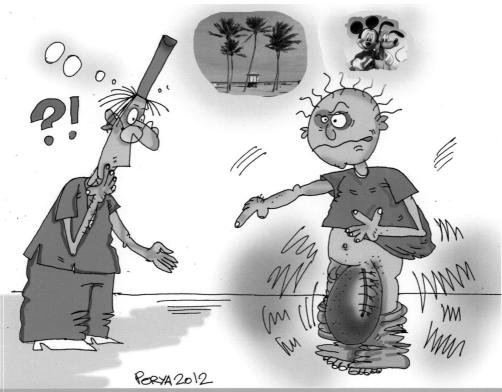

You can judge the worth of a surgeon by the way he does a hernia.

Thomas Fairbank, 1876-1961

Abdominal compartment syndrome after aortic surgery

"Why did I close his abdomen?!"

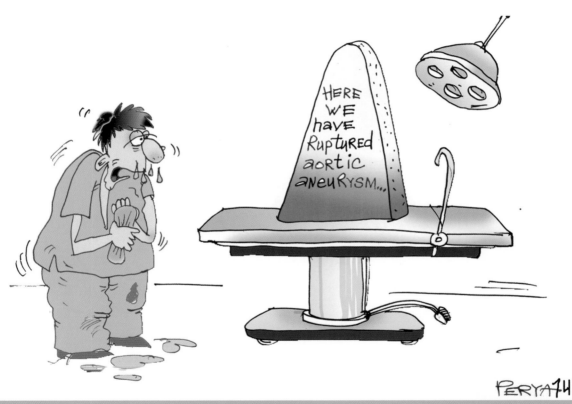

Avoidance of abdominal compartment syndrome is crucial in these physiologically compromised patients in whom any further derangement may be the straw that breaks the camel's back.

Paul N. Rogers

95

Anastomotic leaks

"Operate? Treat conservatively? Ship out?"

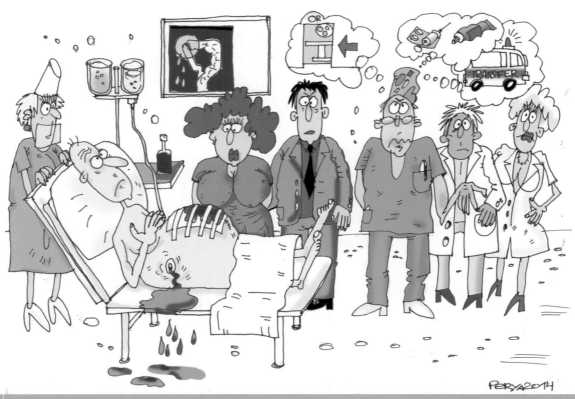

With the exception of exsanguinating postoperative hemorrhage there is nothing that the surgeon fears more than a leaking anastomosis.

MS

Leaking colorectal anastomosis

"Why, for God's sake, did you do an anastomosis in this patient?"

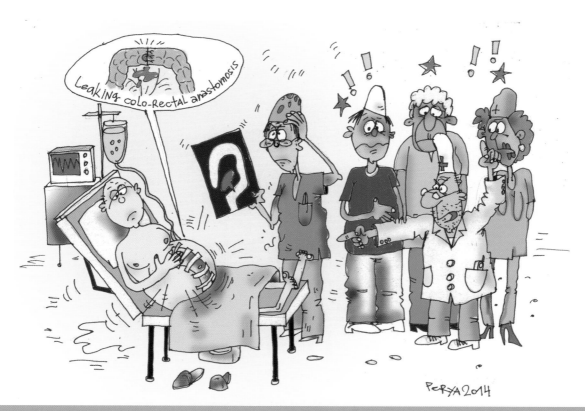

Somebody's leak is a curiosity — one's own leak is a calamity.

The retracted stoma

"Why didn't you do an anastomosis instead?"

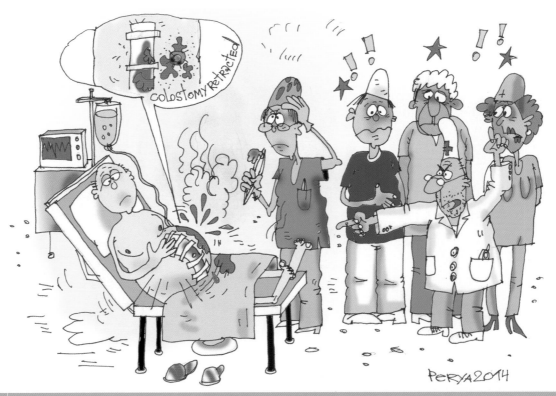

If you think about a colostomy, you should do a colostomy.

Leo A. Gordon

Colonoscopic perforation

"I think that I have lost my way... call the surgeons!"

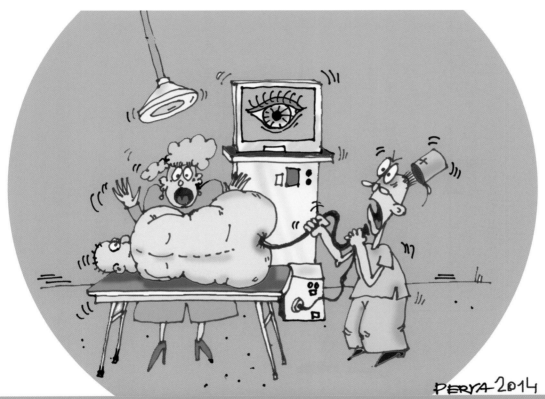

Why are gastroenterologists more imaginative and courageous than us surgeons in employing new and bizarre invasive therapeutic modalities?
Because they have somebody (us) to bail them out!

Eli Mavor

Trocar site hernia

Surgeon: "The good news is that we have cured your biliary dyskinesia!"

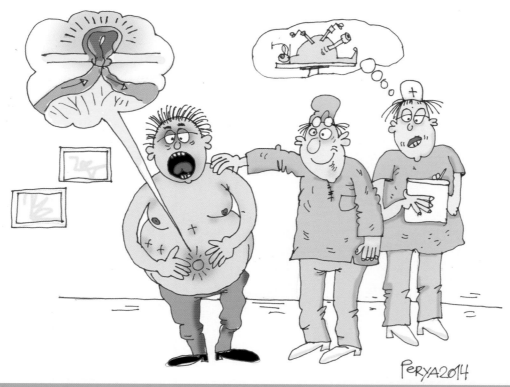

Hernia repairs are like sex... you have to do what works best for you, with the minimum of complaints afterwards.

Angus Maciver

The surgical ostrich syndrome

"Boss, don't worry. I think he is bleeding a little from the incision. We'll pack it and transfuse 2 units of blood. You don't have to come..."

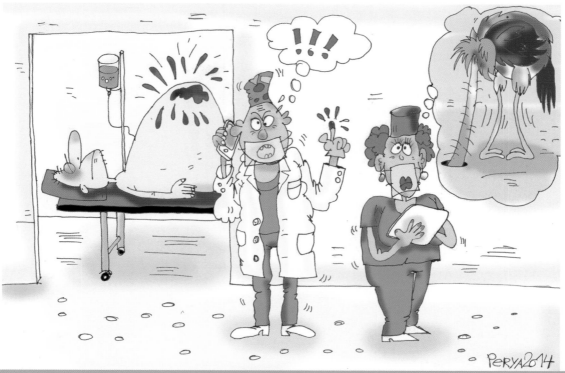

The complication is usually at the primary site of operation unless proven otherwise. Do not behave like a 'surgical ostrich' by ignoring the real problem!

Postop abdominal abscess

"Now that we have color CT it is so easy to diagnose them abscesses…"

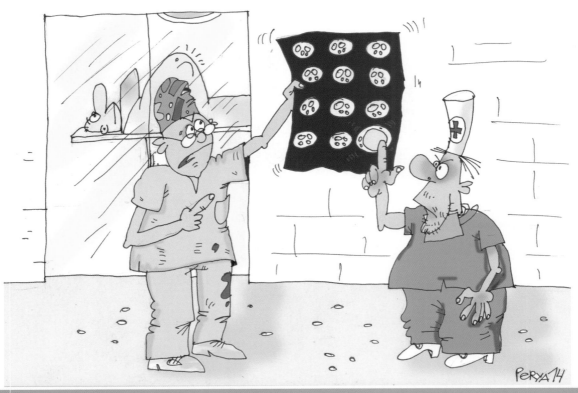

Abdominal abscesses should be drained. When an 'active' source exists it should be dealt with. Antibiotic treatment is of secondary importance.

MS

Wound infection

"This is just a tiny wound abscess — a minor complication... let me lance it for you..."

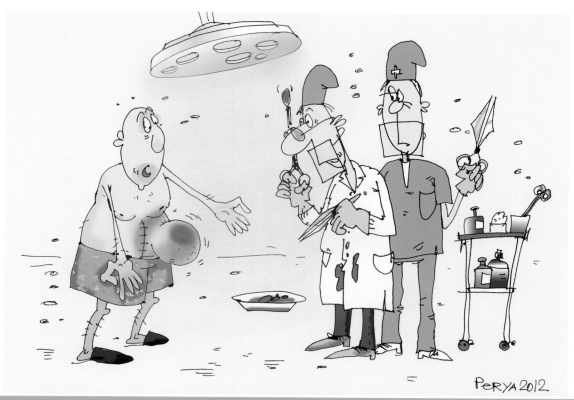

A minor complication is one that happens to somebody else.

Abdominal wall dehiscence

"I can't believe it! I closed him with PDS 1, suture-wound length ratio 4:1..."

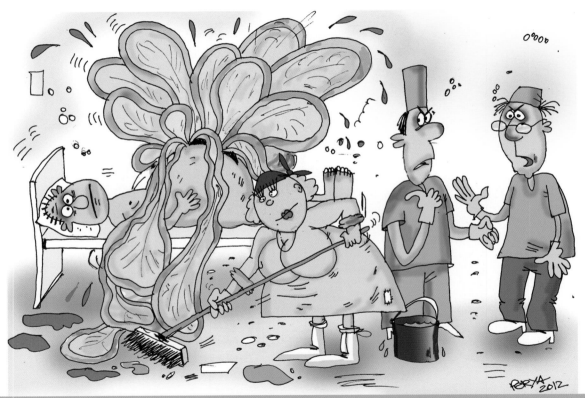

There are few things more embarrassing to a surgeon than the sight of his recently operated patient, his abdomen gaping, and the gut spilling out all around...

MS

Strangulated trocar site hernia

Postop day 3 after laparoscopic cholecystectomy:
Surgeon: "This is ileus, let us try a small enema..."

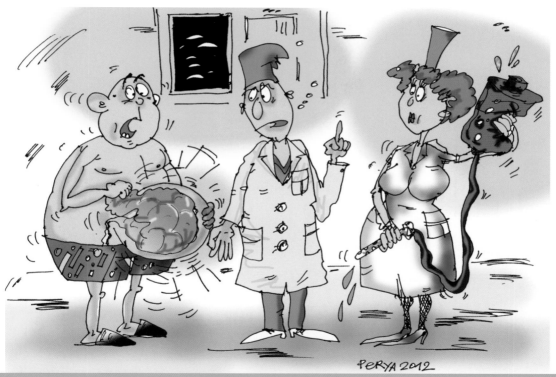

More mistakes are made from want of a proper examination than for any other reason.
Russell John Howard, 1875-1942

Common bile duct injury

"Sir, I thought that this was the cystic duct!"

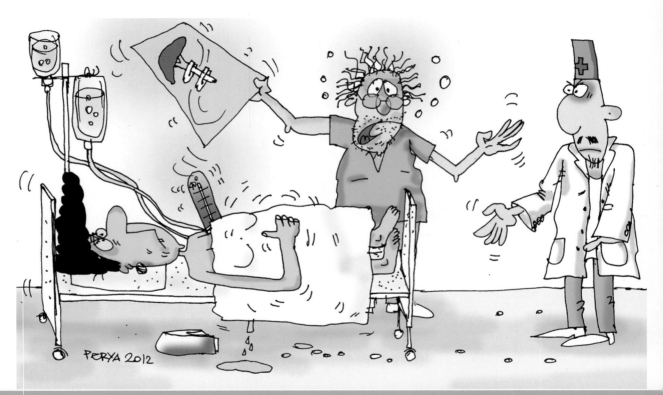

The chief aim of laparoscopic cholecystectomy is not to damage the common bile duct — the secondary aim is to take out the gallbladder.

Kristoffer Lassen

After laparoscopic appendectomy

"Doc, you didn't say that my appendix had perforated into my belly button!"

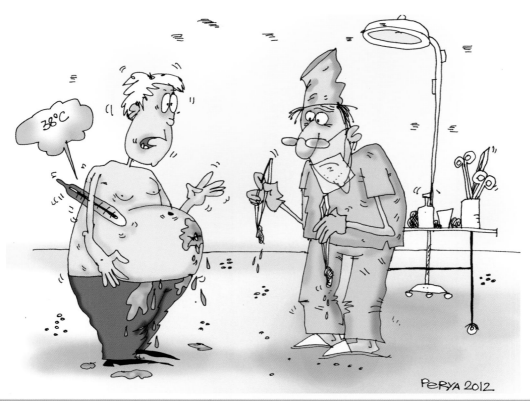

The 'viral' spread of lap appendectomy has increased the spectrum and severity of complications. You won't find it in the <u>biased</u> literature but <u>overall</u> — lap appy is more potentially dangerous than the open one.

Recurrent laryngeal nerve palsy after thyroid surgery

"Nessun dorma, nessun dorma. Can you hear me?"

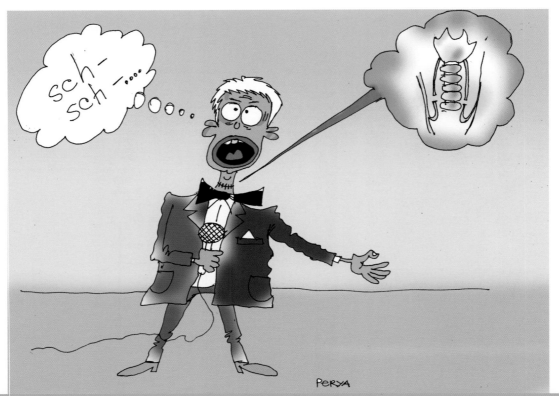

Unilateral recurrent laryngeal nerve damage produces voice changes, but not choking: they graduate in the choir from singing "Ave Maria" to "Old Man River".

David Dent

Limb loss after peripheral arterial surgery

Patient: "Doc, do you think that the aortobifemoral bypass was justified?"
Surgeon: "Absolutely! We managed to save your thighs!"

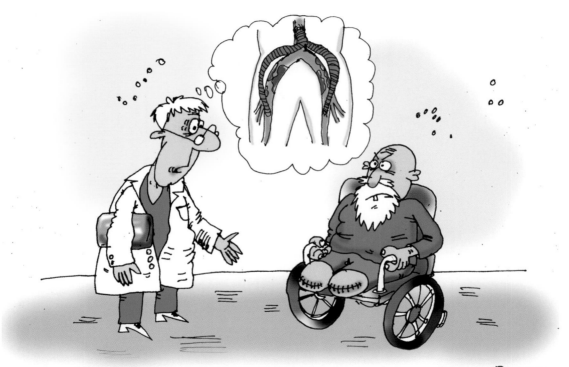

Patients do not need a functioning graft to sit in a wheel chair or lie in bed; an amputation stump would do.

Paul N. Rogers

109

The retained appendix

"Doctor, how is it possible? I had laparoscopic appendectomy at the Mayonnaise Clinic last year!"

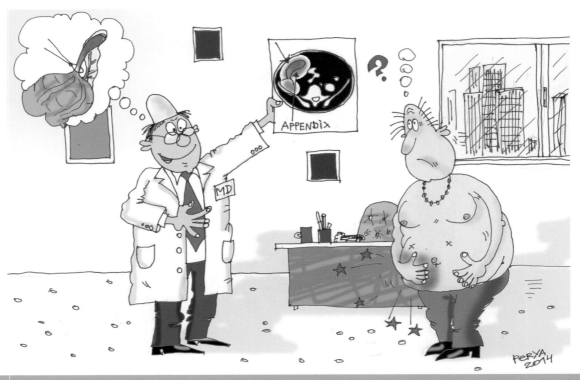

Laparoscopy shares many similarities with the emperor's cloth. If you do not join in the choir of praises you are either stupid or unfit for the job. But someone needs to tell the truth.

Roland Andersson

Oh shit moment

Surgeon: "Oh God, don't pull on the right lobe... we are losing her..."
Assistant: "Sir, you said you need exposure..."

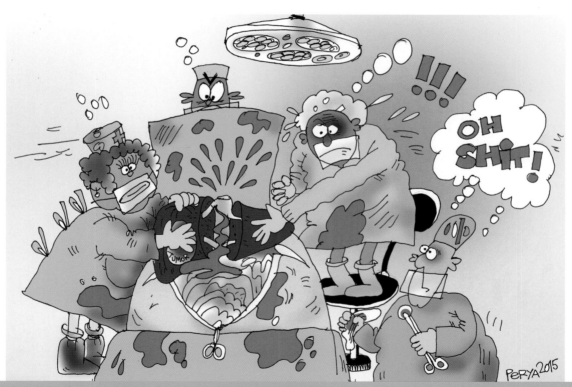

Beware the hemorrhage that has all the blood draining from the surgeon's face.
Stephen Clifforth

The morbidity and mortality conference

"Why didn't you operate? Why did you operate? Why didn't you re-explore? Why was no CT ordered? You've killed him!"

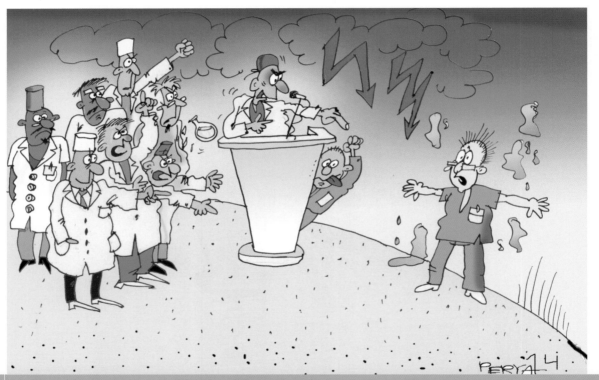

It is either S**T happens or S**T should not have happened. But even if S**T happens it can stink!

MS

6 Miscellaneous

Money talks

The owner of the Rolls: "You have to learn how to bill... for each endoscopy I charge: level 5 consult, diagnostic endoscopy, therapeutic endoscopy and I add a modifier for complexity..."

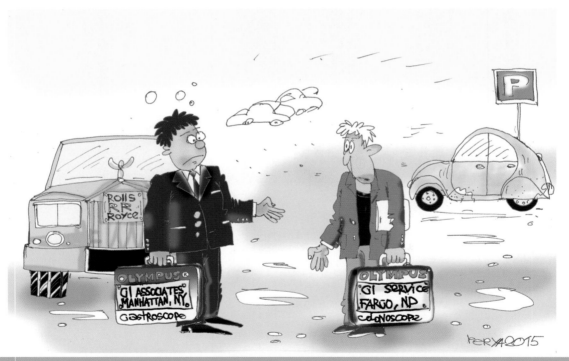

Everyone wants to make a buck out of the medical monster. That is why it costs so much to keep it alive.

Francis D. Moore, 1913-2001

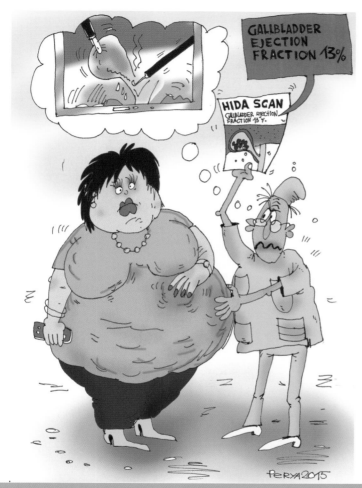

Biliary dyskinesia

Surgeon: "The problem is your lazy gallbladder, we need to take it out!"

Patient: "Is my gallbladder on the left side?"

Cholecystectomy for biliary dyskinesia is an 'American operation' for a 'Made in the USA' alleged disease. This entity is almost unknown elsewhere.

Esophageal foreign body and fishing

"What fish was it? I need the correct bait..."

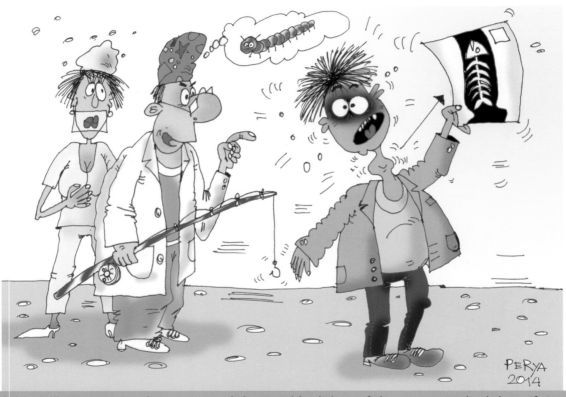

In fishing, like in surgery, there are good days and bad days. If there were no bad days, if everything would go always smoothly — fish biting every day and all day long, and gallbladders popping out within 5 minutes, like a sebaceous cyst — then fishing and surgery would not be as exciting and satisfying. Luckily , however (for the patients), the practice of surgery is a little more predictable than fishing.

MS

Inguinal hernia

"Nice hernia! I can fix it with the laparoscope!"

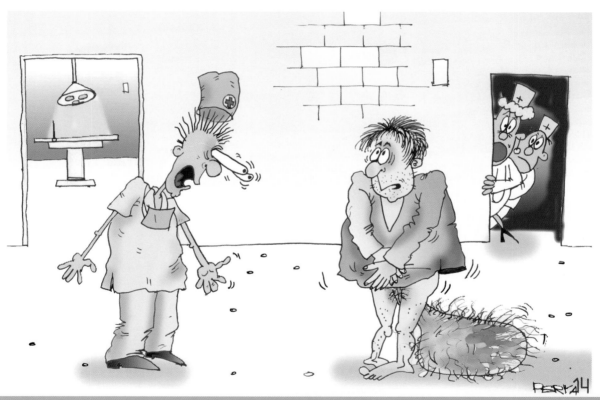

Laparoscopic hernia repair is like going to the center of the Earth to plant a seed near the surface.
Rolando Ramos

Incarcerated ventral hernia

Surgeon: "I'll reduce the hernia, insert mesh... 15 minutes..."
Medical student: "Sir, did you ask for a CT?"

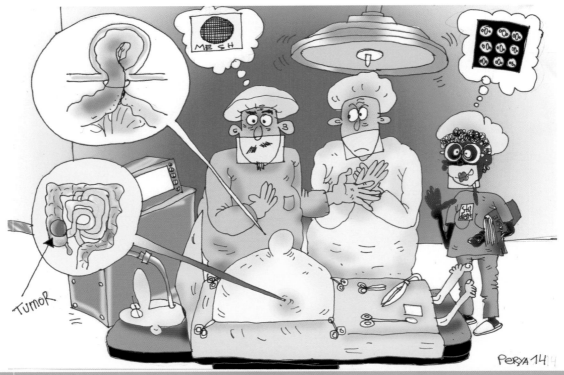

Distinguish between intestinal obstruction <u>caused</u> by the incisional hernia or simply <u>associated</u> with it!

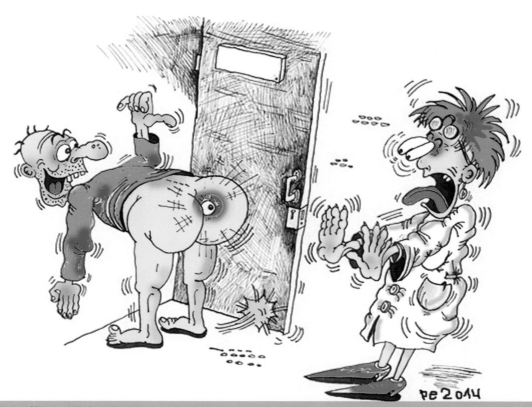

Anal pain

"Pain in the ass!"

We suffer and die through the defects that arise in our sewerage and drainage systems.
William A. Lane, 1856-1943

On the liver transplant list

"He's doing fine for somebody on the transplant list!"

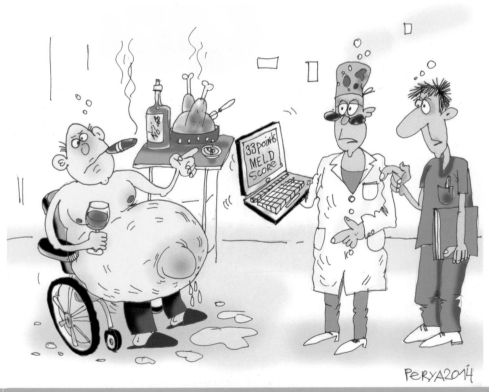

Liver transplantation (in alcoholics) was the ultimate sobering experience.

Thomas Starzl

The acute scrotum

"Doc, she is driving me nuts!" Bradley Morris
"He was having too big a ball with the wrong girl..." Barry Alexander
"A blank exploration is better than a black testis." Hafez Serhal

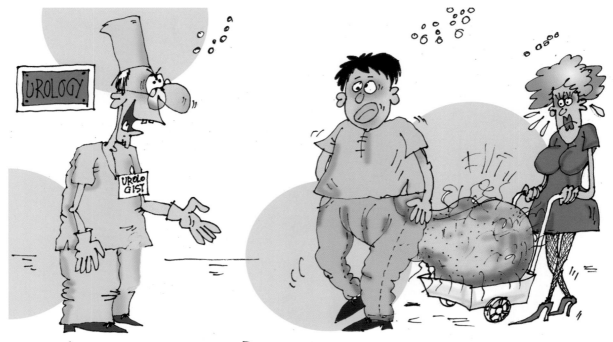

To the urologist the 'acute scrotum' is the equivalent to the general surgeon's 'acute abdomen'.

Pediatric surgery

Surgeon: "I'm a pediatric surgeon... not bariatric!"
Parents: "Betty is five years old, we think it's biliary dyskinesia."
Surgeon: "What were you feeding her?"

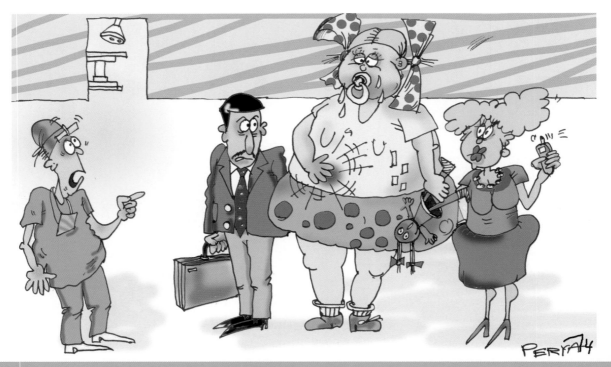

High fructose corn syrup is poisoning America!

Wound care with honey

"Welcome to my center of HONEY wound management!"

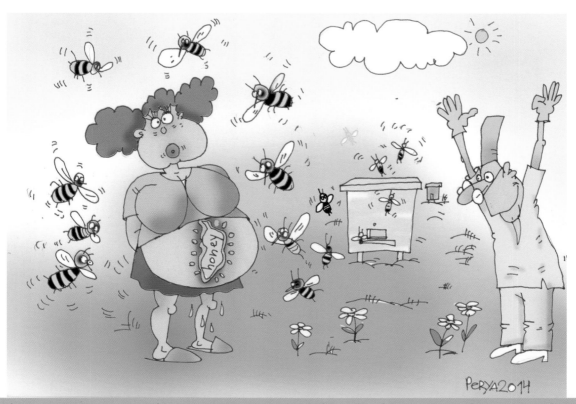

If thou examinest a man having a gaping wound thou shouldst treat it afterward with grease, honey, (and) lint every day, until he recovers.

Edwin Smith Papyrus, written in Egypt, ~3000 years ago

Colonoscopy

"This is clearly a cancer in the cecum — there is no need to tattoo it..."

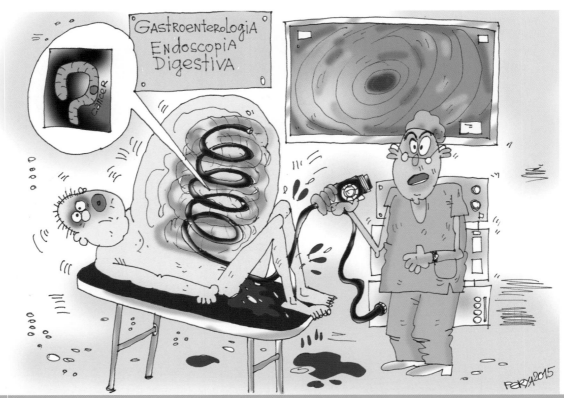

I know when the colonoscope is in the rectum and the ileum but ensuring any location anywhere else in the colon is a crapshoot.

Jon Efron

Intensive care unit

"Guys, what other tubes or lines have we forgotten to insert?"

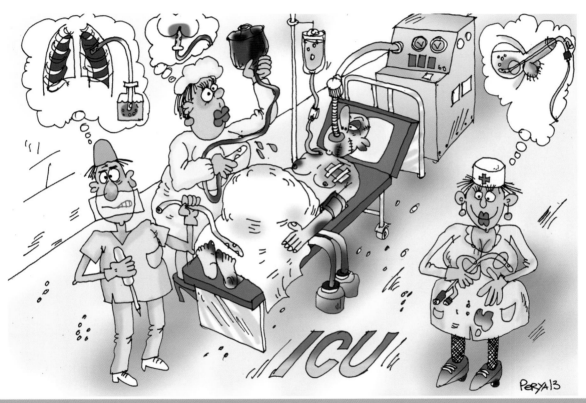

This is the reality of intensive care: at any point, we are as apt to harm as we are to heal.

Atul Gawande

Portal hypertension

Surgeon: "Not sure which portocaval shunt he needs? Mesocaval? Distal splenorenal?"
Resident: "But Sir, he is Child's C!"

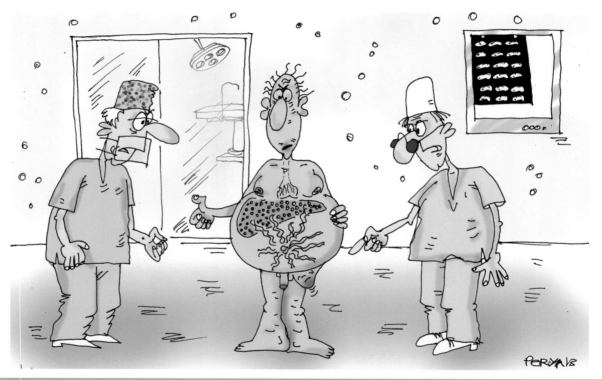

Child C patients have a short life expectancy — unless transplanted — and they should only be operated upon if there is no other option and should be clearly informed about their high mortality risk.

Erik Schadde

Operating on children

Nurse: "He plays Nintendo, eh?"
Anesthetist: "Yep. Unfortunately they don't read books these days."

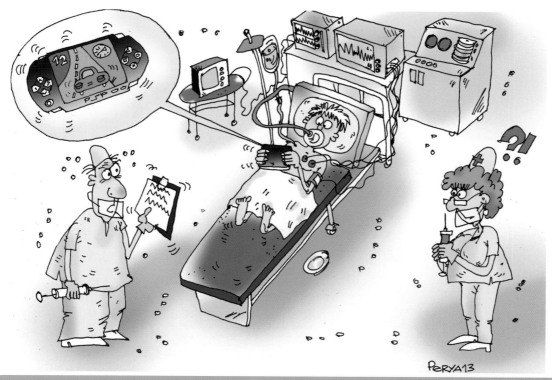

Let us try and make the ordeal of operation on children as uneventful as possible so they can play with their toys on the way to the OR and as soon as possible after waking up from anesthesia!
Graeme Pitcher

Urology

Five days after a laparoscopic R hemicolectomy:
Wife: "What's that? Have you spilled beer on your pyjamas?"
Husband: "I don't know… it smells like urine… this is where they had left a drain."

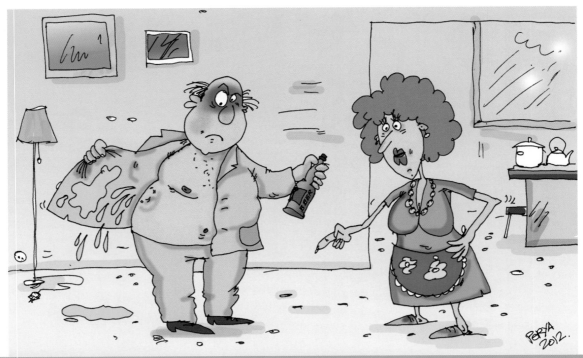

Treat the urinary system the same as your garden hose pipe: as the water goes in, it should go out; if not then fix or dislodge or stent and if desperate just drain and try again later.

MS

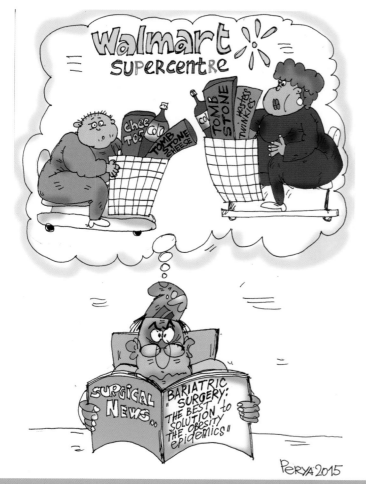

Morbid obesity

"In the USA alone there are 15.5 million people with a BMI of >40. Can we operate on all of them?"

Fat people don't need surgery. They need to not put food in their mouths.

Mastectomy vs. lumpectomy

Patient: "I want this breast completely off."
Surgeon: "Sorry Mam, but my mastectomy/lumpectomy rate is higher than the national average... one more mastectomy and I'll lose my breast privileges."

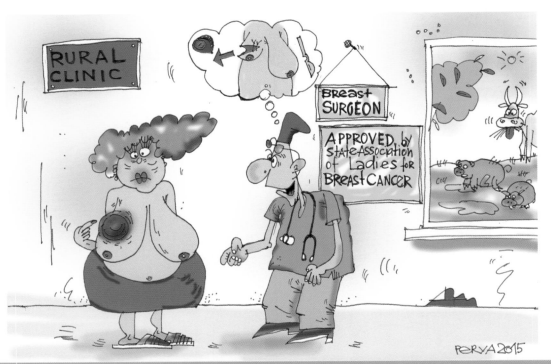

Breast doctors are usually called Monica or Kimberley, having a web site with help page, a clinic with flowers, plants and statuary, a public grouping raising money, and the shrill insinuation at large meetings that XYs were mutilating women and this must stop!

David Dent

Clinical guidelines

"This is the abbreviated version of our simplified guidelines. Now let us go to page 40…"

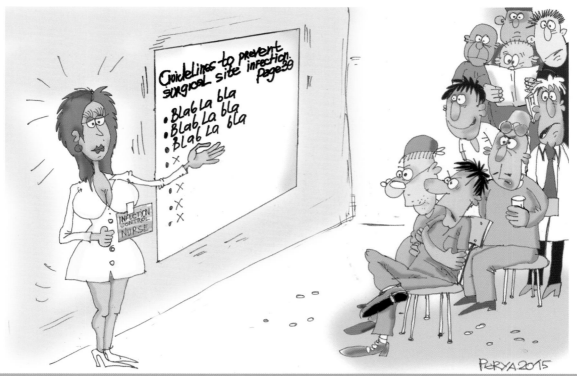

The good thing about 'guidelines' is that there are so many to choose from…

Ascending cholangitis

"The urine is also dark... what do you call that triad? Charcoal?"

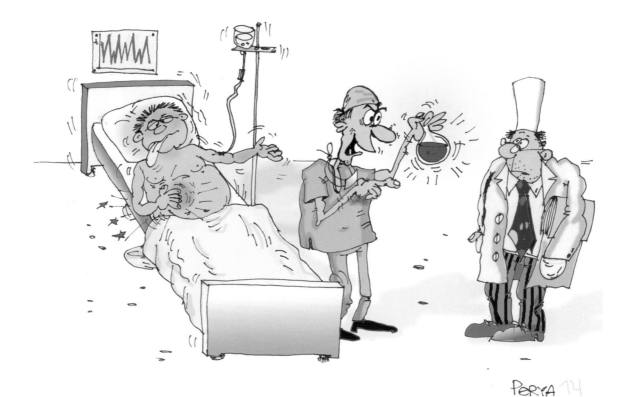

Charcot triad for ascending cholangitis: right upper quadrant pain, jaundice, and fever.
Jean-Martin Charcot, 1825-1893

Pre-operative optimization

"We need to hydrate you a little... so you will tolerate the blood loss."

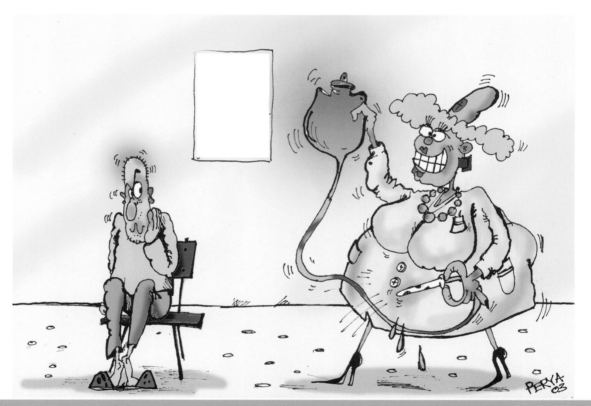

The preparation of the patient for surgery is as crucial as the operation itself.

SURGINET

"Guys, what should I do?"

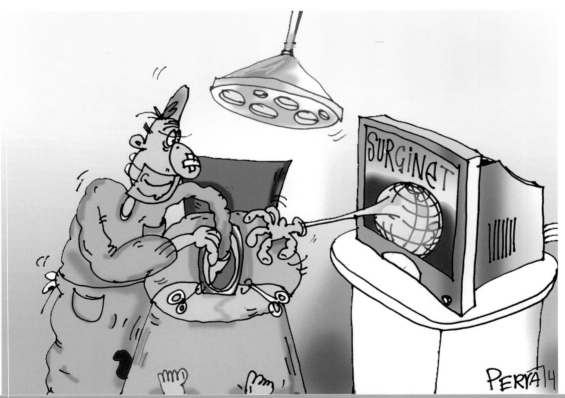

SURGINET is the largest online, international discussion forum for general surgeons. To subscribe please email me at mosheschein@gmail.com.

MS

Index